THE ULTIMATE GUIDE TO BETTER SKIN

# BEAUTIFUL SKIN REVEALED

REAL PATIENTS AND THEIR STORIES

BY PAUL M. FRIEDMAN, MD

JOY H. KUNISHIGE, MD AND KRISTEL D. POLDER, MD

**PUBLISHED BY**
NewBeauty® Magazine
Sandow Media
3731 NW 8th Avenue | Boca Raton, FL 33458
www.newbeauty.com


**LIBRARY OF CONGRESS CONTROL NUMBER** 2010921189

**ISBN** 978-0-9800398-2-5


Printed in China

First Edition | March 2010
10 9 8 7 6 5 4 3 2 1

# DEDICATIONS

**To my patients** for their inspiration and for revealing
their inner and outer beauty in order to help others.

**To my loving and supportive parents,**
Irving and Diane Friedman.

**To my siblings,** Robin H. Friedman-Musicante, MD,
and Edward S. Friedman, MD for believing in me.

**To Roy G. Geronemus, MD, Leonard H. Goldberg, MD, Tina S. Alster, MD,
and Frederic S. Brandt, MD** for their friendship and mentorship.

**To Ronald P. Rapini, MD, Madeline A. Duvic, MD, and the faculty and residents**
at the University of Texas Medical School at Houston Department of Dermatology
for their encouragement and support.

**To my teachers in medicine,** the faculty at the NYU Medical Center
Department of Dermatology, Washington University School of Medicine
Internal Medicine Department, and University of Tennessee School of Medicine.

**To Sergio A. Musicante, MD, Timothy H. Eidson, MD,
and Scott Kramer** for their friendship.

**To my nieces and nephews,** Meryl, Robbie, Jacob, Abie, and Mia Molly
for teaching me the truly important things in life.

# ACKNOWLEDGEMENTS

| | |
|---|---|
| co-author | Joy H. Kunishige, MD |
| contributing author and editor | Kristel D. Polder, MD |
| distributor | Publishers Group West |
| editors | Robin H. Friedman-Musicante, MD |
| | Dawn Dorsey, Meryl Musicante, Aly Walansky |
| reviewers | Roy G. Geronemus, MD; Tina S. Alster, MD; Fredric S. Brandt, MD |
| testimonials | Denise K. Marquez, PA |
| creative consultant | Nancy Flores |
| photography | Julie Soefer |
| additional photography | Mariae Bui, Raheem Osanyin (Lucy and Veronica) |
| hair and makeup | Edward Sanchez |
| additional hair and makeup | Mariel Munoz |
| cover design | Allyson Lack |
| consultants | Anne Akers, Anja Krammer, Elizabeth Gammon, PhD |
| | Jessica Yadegar, Erika Abrahamsson, Joanna Kornfeld |
| dermsurgery laser center | Leonard H. Goldberg, MD; Denise K. Marquez, PA, Silvia Villareal, RN |
| | Angel Ozaeta, MA, Joseph Villabroza, MA, Natasha Migueles, MA |
| | Lisa Kandler, MA, Violet Plata, Tracy M. Katz, MD |
| assistants | Sarah Seitz, Kris Cunningham, Jennifer M. Landau |
| photoshoot locations | Brian S. Spack |
| counsel | Tamera H. Bennett, Paul J. Friedman, Sanford L. Dow |
| | Scott A. Kramer, Michael A. Harvey |

THE ULTIMATE GUIDE TO BETTER SKIN

# BEAUTIFUL SKIN REVEALED

REAL PATIENTS AND THEIR STORIES

BY PAUL M. FRIEDMAN, MD

JOY H. KUNISHIGE, MD AND KRISTEL D. POLDER, MD

## TABLE OF CONTENTS

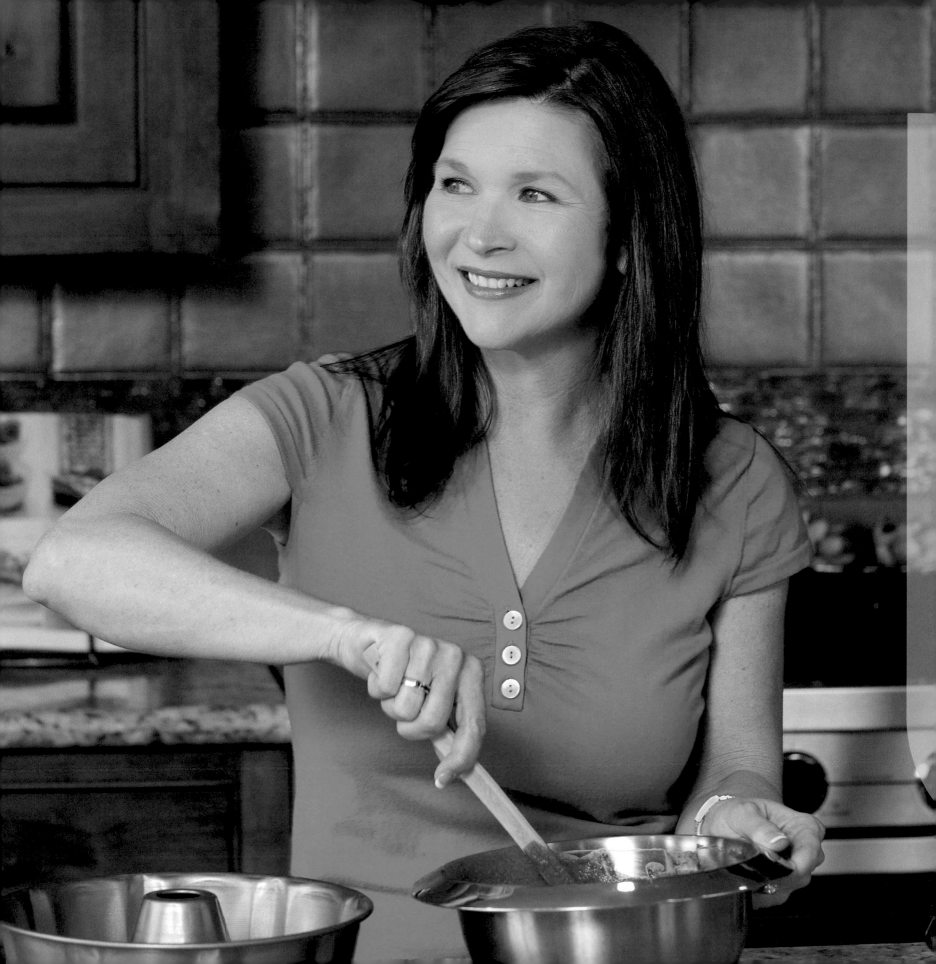

# CHAPTER 1

# COMPLEXION

> " For about nine years,
> I had a brown sun spot on my forehead,
> RIGHT BETWEEN MY EYEBROWS." – *Cathey, 45*

Uneven complexion may be the number-one complaint heard by dermatologists. While looking carefully at your face, pay attention to your skin's overall composition. Would you say your skin color seems splotchy, with flat, tan freckles or brown spots dotting the cheeks? Or is your skin texture dull and slightly gray? Discolorations and textural irregularities can rob your complexion of its inherent brightness—at any age.

# Why it occurs

THERE ARE TWO TYPES OF SKIN AGING: INTRINSIC AGING FROM TIME AND GENETICS, AND EXTRINSIC AGING CAUSED PRIMARILY BY THE SUN. Other extrinsic factors are smoking, repeated facial expressions, sleeping position, and gravity. How and why does skin change over time?

If you imagine skin cells as a brick wall, then ceramides—a pasty element that helps retain moisture—serve as the mortar between each brick. At age 20, our body's ability to make ceramides starts to wane, and over the years, the result is dry, flaky skin. Skin cells don't naturally exfoliate, making the topmost layer of the skin thick. Light hitting this uneven and thick skin bounces back chaotically so the skin appears dull. Inner glow is not really from the inside; it is light reflecting off the outside.

Collagen is a key component in youthful skin. Over time, we make less collagen and elastic fibers, so skin has less recoil, like a used rubber band. As we age, there is also less underlying fat, or volume. Reduced underlying volume results in loose, saggy skin.

It was once assumed that aging was skin's biggest enemy, but we now know environmental factors play a key role. The effects of the sun are huge! Sun breaks down our collagen and elastic fibers. The broken fibers clump together, creating knots of collagen. The knots result in a bumpy skin surface resembling leather. Scientists and physicians studying biopsy specimens under the microscope can actually estimate the age and cumulative sun exposure of a patient by observing the amount of clumped collagen and elastic fibers.

Sun-worshipers, beware. Over time your skin will compensate to protect itself by producing melanin. More melanin means more pigment (sun spots and brown spots), which are evidence of photodamage. Unusually high sun exposure over a long period of time can result in your apparent "age" being off by as much as 20 years!

## PATIENT T!P

Put a translucent powder with SPF 30 in your purse and touch up throughout the day to maintain sun protection.

# " Cathey's story

**AGE:** 45
**CONCERN:** SUN SPOTS
**TREATMENT:** 694-NM Q-SWITCHED RUBY LASER
**NUMBER OF TREATMENTS:** 1
**DOWNTIME:** 2–3 DAYS MINIMAL CRUSTING; 1 WEEK MINIMAL REDNESS

**BEFORE**

**AFTER**

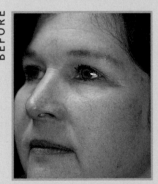

For about nine years, I had a brown sun spot on my forehead, right between my eyebrows. It bothered me because I have very fair skin, so to me, this made the brown spot stand out more than normal. My regular dermatologist kept telling me that nothing could really be done. She said she could 'freeze' it off but that this might result in a white spot. The white spot seemed worse than having the brown sun spot, so I didn't do anything. Eventually, my dermatologist referred me to a laser specialist.

The Q-switched ruby laser was used to treat my forehead sun spot, as well as other smaller sun spots on my cheeks and one on my temple. The procedure didn't hurt at all and was over in about five or 10 minutes. The brown spots turned very dark at first, almost black. This worried me, but I knew it was supposed to do that. I treated the spots daily with Aquaphor and used bandages for about eight days to keep the spots out of the sun. After eight days, the dark spots sloughed off while I was showering, and they were gone. I continued (and still do) to cover the spots with SPF 45 sunscreen.

Everything is great now. I have no sun spots! I was lucky because it worked after just one treatment—sometimes it takes two or three times to achieve good results. Even if another treatment becomes necessary, I would not hesitate to do it."

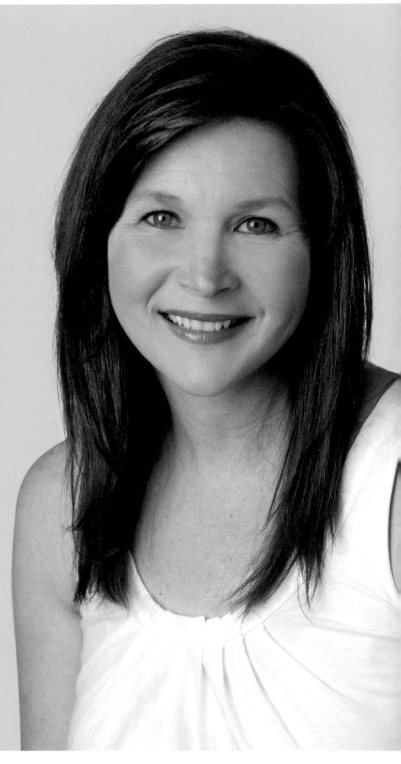

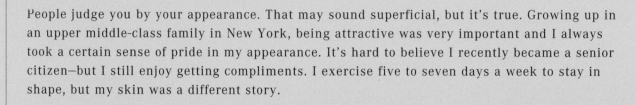

# Carole's story

**AGE:** 66
**CONCERN:** FACIAL REDNESS, UNEVEN SKIN TONE, AND PIGMENT DISCOLORATION
**TREATMENT:** VBEAM LASER, FRAXEL RE:STORE LASER
**NUMBER OF TREATMENTS:** 4 FRAXEL, 8 VBEAM
**DOWNTIME:** 3–4 DAYS

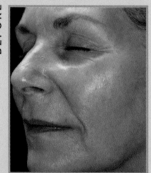

BEFORE

AFTER

People judge you by your appearance. That may sound superficial, but it's true. Growing up in an upper middle-class family in New York, being attractive was very important and I always took a certain sense of pride in my appearance. It's hard to believe I recently became a senior citizen—but I still enjoy getting compliments. I exercise five to seven days a week to stay in shape, but my skin was a different story.

All the years of sun damage finally caught up with me. Every time I looked in the mirror I found a new brown splotch or another patch of redness. I tried creams, gels, ointments, peels and injections—the problems only seemed to get worse. I was tired of wearing layers of makeup every day to camouflage my skin. I wanted my skin to be one color again. The doctor recommended laser treatments, assuring me they would make a profound difference in my appearance. I was skeptical.

After four Fraxel re:store™ and eight VBeam® Perfecta laser treatments, the texture of my skin dramatically improved. My skin actually glows, and the discoloration and blotchy red patches are almost completely faded. A nice bonus is my skin is also firmer.

Today, instead of using heavy foundation, I now apply powder with a brush. That's it. My husband recently said I look better without makeup. Now, whether I am at the health club, shopping, or out with my grandchildren, I have a renewed sense of confidence in my appearance. Those who know me think I had a facelift or some other 'work' done. No more potions and lotions for me. Laser treatments have brought back the 'glow' I thought I left behind in my youth."

## PATIENT T!P

Fraxel laser treatments can sting a little, but only during the procedure. Afterward, try cooling your face with a bag of frozen peas or ice packs.

## A conversation
## with the doctor

BLOTCHINESS IS A COMMON COMPLAINT. Sunblock is the answer, but once the damage is done, peels or lasers are a great way to erase pigment.

Everyone is trying to achieve that elusive "glow," but the glow is nothing more than a reflection of light bouncing off your skin. Outer glow can be yours. Think of a baby's skin. It has a thin, even top layer so light bounces off, which is perceived as being youthful and fresh. As we age, skin cells stay packed on top like a pebbly surface creating a duller impression.

Studies have shown that texture and pigment are subconsciously interpreted as indicators of age. Chemical peels and some lasers can level this surface out. Non-ablative lasers heat skin beneath the surface, causing collagen remodeling. Stimulating new collagen growth results in skin feeling firmer. You get a bit of tightening and toning effect. Maintenance includes touch-ups every six to 12 months. It's important to use sunblock daily, or your skin will revert to its former condition.

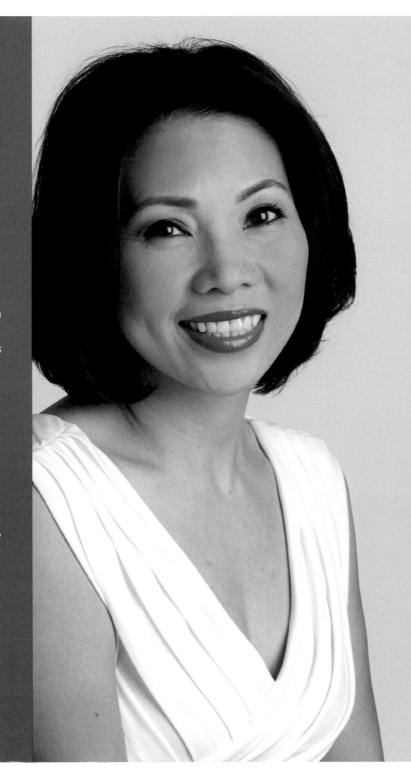

# Mani

AGE: 38

CONCERN: SUN SPOTS

TREATMENT: 532-NM

Q-SWITCHED ND:YAG LASER

NUMBER OF TREATMENTS: 2

DOWNTIME: 2-3 DAYS

MINIMAL CRUSTING;

1 WEEK MINIMAL REDNESS

BEFORE
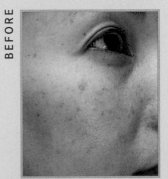

AFTER
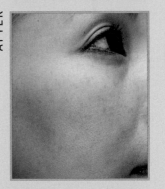

# What to expect
## (time, cost, recovery, permanence, risk)

REMEMBER EVERY FACE IS AN AGING FACE...AND SKIN DOES NOT STOP AT THE JAW LINE. Your skin's condition is part DNA (intrinsic) and part environment (extrinsic). The latter is in your control. The former can be addressed by familiarizing yourself with the multitude of treatments and preventative measures available and choosing what is best for you.

| Procedure | Time | Approx. cost per treatment* | Treatments |
|---|---|---|---|
| Microdermabrasion crystals physically exfoliate a few cells from the top layer of skin for quick brightening | 15 minutes | $150 | 3–6 |
| Superficial chemical peel (i.e. 15% trichloroacetic acid peel or glycolic peel) solution dissolves few cells from top layer for a quick, fresh glow | 10 minutes | $150 | 3 |
| Medium-depth chemical peel (i.e. Jessner's + 30% trichloroacetic acid peel) solution removes variable layers of skin to lighten brown spots and soften fine lines | 20 minutes | $300 | 1–2 |
| Q-switched lasers heat and break up pigment within the skin | 30 minutes for topical anesthesia, 10 minutes for procedure | $400–$600 | 1–2 |
| Fractional non-ablative technology (i.e. Fraxel re:store™, Lux 1540™) uses miniscule columns of light to heat the skin beneath the surface to encourage collagen remodeling | 1 hour for topical anesthesia, 30 minutes for laser treatment | $1,000 | 3–5 |
| Fractional ablative resurfacing (i.e. Fraxel re:pair®, Lux 2940™) uses tiny columns of light to partially remove surface skin | 1 hour for anesthesia, 1 hour for procedure | $4,000–$5,000 | 1–2 |

*Cost varies widely from practice to practice, and geographically. Costs are very approximate estimates at time of publication.

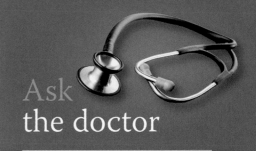

Ask
the doctor

### WHAT CONDITIONS CAN FRACTIONATED NON-ABLATIVE LASERS TREAT?

Fractionated non-ablative lasers can be used to effectively treat a number of conditions, including photoaging, fine lines, crepiness, melasma, irregular pigmentation, and enlarged pores. An additional advantage of this technology is that it can safely be used to treat areas other than the face, such as the neck, chest and hands. These areas were difficult to treat with previous resurfacing techniques because of the risk of scarring. Fractionated lasers can also be used on all skin types.

Patients are often concerned about the amount of discomfort involved. The good news is that the newer non-ablative fractional lasers are quite tolerable with topical anesthetic. Keep in mind, however, that the further away from the face, the longer the healing process. Redness may persist on the neck, chest and hands for several days following treatment.

| Recovery | Permanence | Risks |
|---|---|---|
| Immediately ready for work | May need touch-up treatment every 1–3 months | None |
| Immediately ready for work, very mild peeling 3–7 days after procedure | May need touch-up peel every 2-3 months | Dark or light spots |
| 5 days no work, then 3 days redness | Permanent improvement, may desire another treatment in 1 year | Dark or light spots, herpes simplex reactivation, rarely other infection |
| Areas treated will turn white and swelling may occur following treatment. White lesion will then darken, forming a scab that will fall off in 7-10 days. | May desire touch-up treatment every 6 months | Dark or light spots uncommon, variable response |
| Areas treated will have redness and swelling for a few days. May cover with makeup. | Variable, may desire touch-up treatment in 6 months. Sun exposure will bring dark spots back. | Dark or light spots, herpes simplex reactivation |
| 5-7 days no work, areas treated will have redness for up to a month and swelling for a week after treatment. Pinpoint bleeding and oozing may occur for 48 hours. | Permanent, some benefit from one additional treatment | Dark spots, herpes simplex reactivation, infection which can cause scarring |

"I feel and look 10 years younger, and I don't have to shy away from the camera or turn my head to hide my sun spots."

– Mani, 38

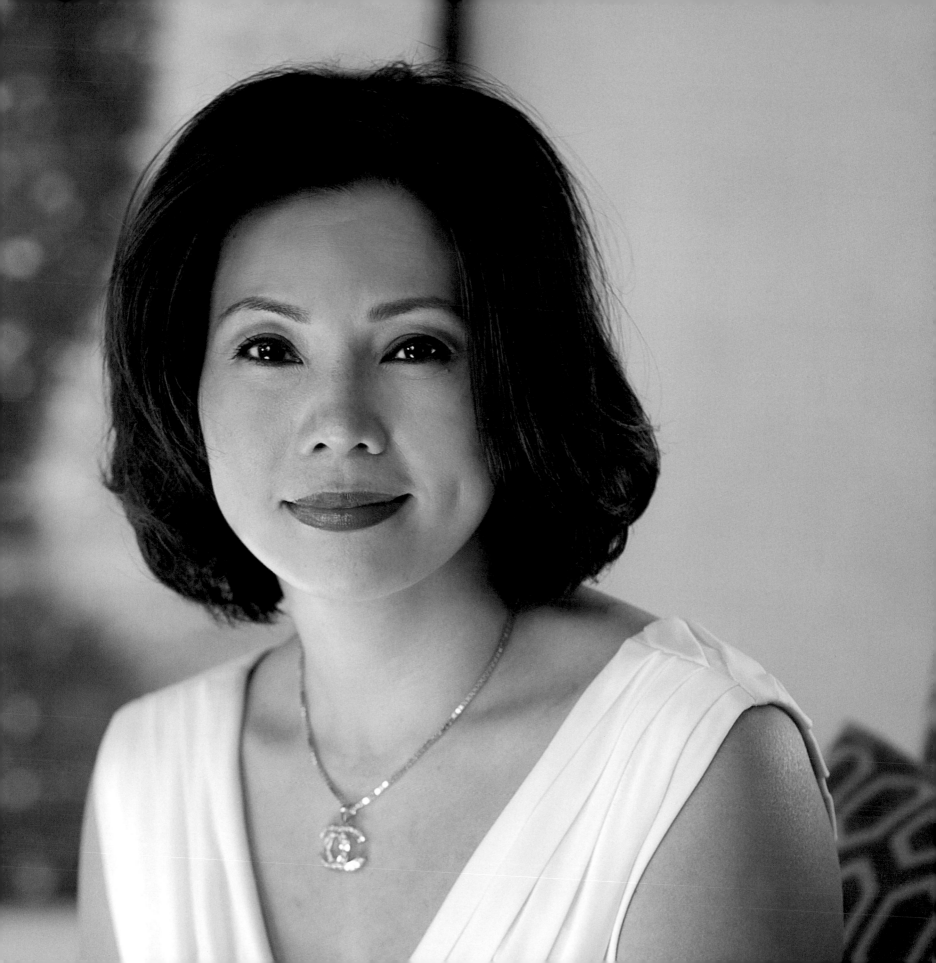

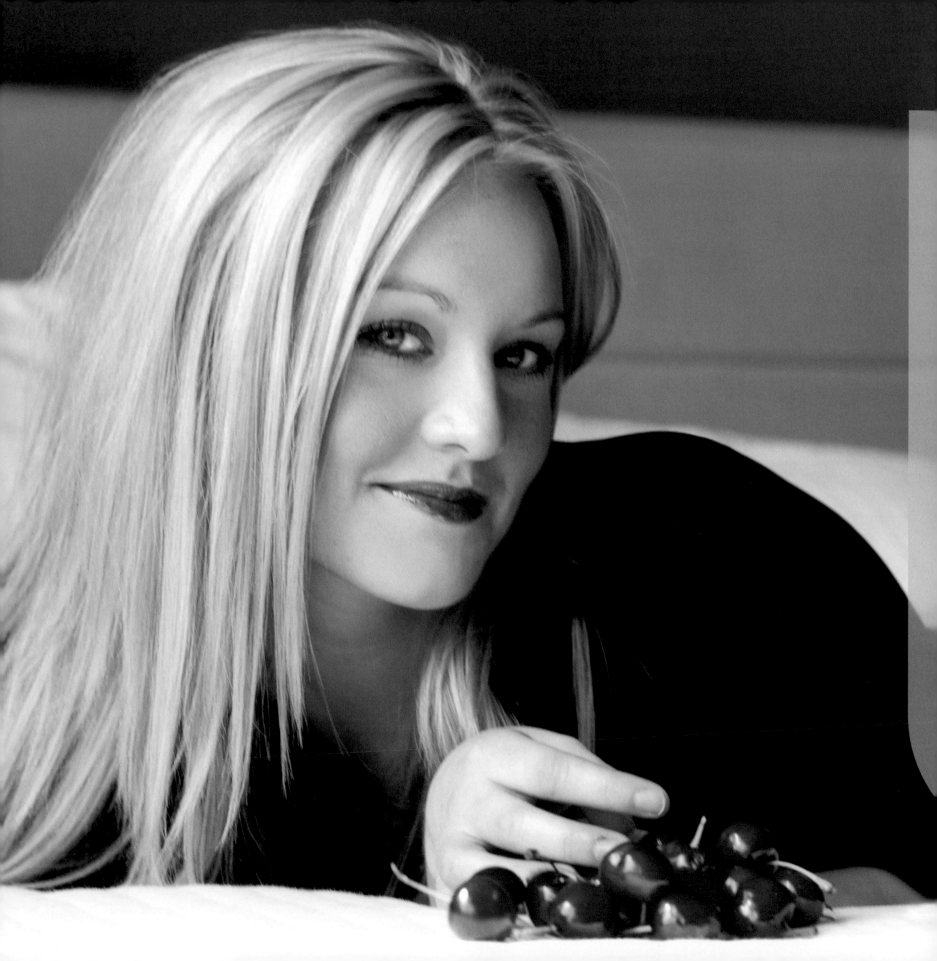

# ACNE

# CHAPTER 2

> " The severe acne I struggled with for 11 years LEFT ME WITH PHYSICAL AND EMOTIONAL SCARRING."
>
> – Ashley, 23

It may surprise you to learn that 1 in 5 adults between the ages of 25 and 44 experiences acne. In fact, some find their acne is worse in adulthood than it was during puberty. Permanent facial scars or changes in skin color serve as constant physical reminders, and the emotional toll on self-esteem and overall confidence are deeply felt—even among adults. The good news is there are new treatments designed to easily and effectively help adults who are concerned about minimizing scars and getting their acne under control.

# Ashley's story

As a public relations professional, I want to look as good on the outside as I feel on the inside. In this industry, it's always important to put your best face forward. The severe acne I struggled with for 11 years left me with physical and emotional scarring. Whether I was meeting a corporate client or attending a social event, I could NEVER walk out of the house without layers of makeup on my face. It took dozens of different types of creams, antibiotics, and even two rounds of Accutane before my acne was mildly under control. Fortunately, I had an excellent (and very patient) dermatologist who eventually referred me to a laser specialist to see what could be done about my scars. I met with the doctor and brought my last ounce of hope.

Several treatments of the Fraxel re:store laser were recommended. After only two treatments, the red pigment in my scars had disappeared! I tossed out my expensive makeup and only held onto the bare essentials after my fourth treatment. Today, I am officially out of hiding. I don't have to put on a mask just to walk the dogs. It's liberating. As a PR person, I'm thinking of becoming a spokeswoman for Fraxel. It has made a big impact on my quality of life."

AGE: 23
CONCERN: ACNE SCARRING
TREATMENT: FRAXEL RE:STORE LASER
NUMBER OF TREATMENTS: 5
DOWNTIME: 2-3 DAYS

BEFORE

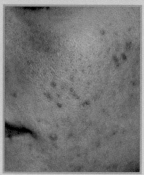

AFTER

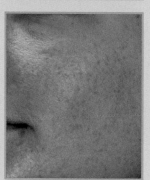

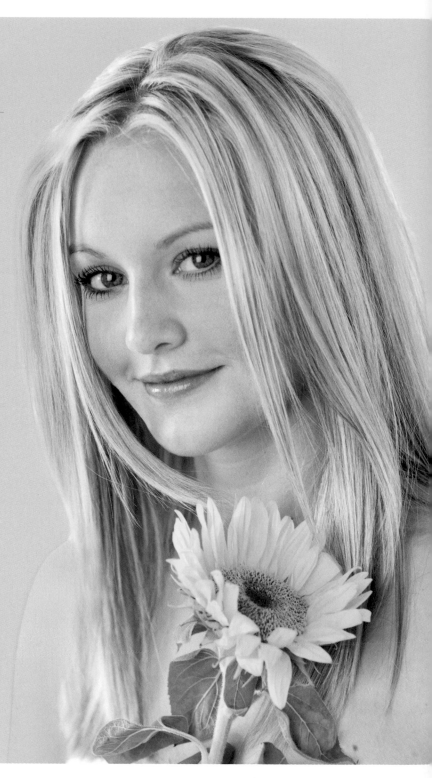

# Why it occurs

NEARLY EVERYBODY THINKS THAT ACNE RESULTS FROM POOR HYGIENE OR AN UNHEALTHY DIET. That's just not accurate. Adult and teen acne are caused by a combination of several factors: genetics, hormones leading to excess oil secretion, faulty closing of the hair duct, and bacteria. Although the precise reason for acne among adults remains unknown, blockages of bacteria and oil can build, leading to adult acne problems, including pimples, inflammation, cysts, and scarring. Adult acne most often appears on the face; however, it can appear on the arms, legs, buttocks, and torso. Contributing factors include side effects from certain medications, occlusive cosmetic products, excessive sweating, stress, pregnancy, and menopause.

Acne at any age starts with occlusion of the hair follicle. Occlusion is caused by skin cells that don't fall off as they should. Even though the top of the hair follicle opening is blocked, the sebaceous gland continues to do its job and secrete sebum into the hair follicle. When the hair follicle is plugged with the trapped sebum, doctors call it a comedone, also known as a whitehead or blackhead. The only difference between a blackhead and a whitehead is that the former has an opening to the surface and is exposed to air turning the contents dark. The latter is closed, but often ruptures—either spontaneously or through tampering—leading to redness, infection, and the papules, pustules, nodules, and cysts of acne.

## The take-home point

It's difficult, but try not to pick your acne. Picking just pushes the inflammation deeper and causes the follicle to rupture, turning simple clogged follicles into inflamed red and angry acne! Tampering increases your risk for scarring.

# Today's treatment options

THERE ARE MANY TOPICAL, ORAL, PHYSICAL, AND NEWLY INTRODUCED LASER TREATMENTS FOR ACNE. This is one disease process medicine and science can correct. Acne scars, however, have limited treatment choices: surgical excision or subscision, injection of dermal fillers, or laser therapy. The laser systems commonly used for acne scarring are: 1450-nm diode, 1320-nm Nd:YAG, fractionated photothermolysis, carbon dioxide, and erbium:YAG.

The foundation of any treatment regimen involves a topical retinoid. The brand names you may recognize are Retin A, Differin, or Tazorac. Retinoids regulate skin turnover and make the skin cells less sticky. Topical and oral antibiotics help reduce inflammation. Acne in women can be treated by regulating hormone levels with oral contraceptives or spironolactone. When acne is severe, Accutane (a brand name isotretinoin) can be prescribed. Accutane is highly regulated by the government, primarily because of the risk of birth defects. Retinoids taken either orally or topically can improve overall skin condition, but do nothing to improve scars.

**Note:** *Roche recalled Accutane from the market in June 2009. Accutane is an isotretinoin and is currently available as Claravis, Sotret, or Amnesteem.*

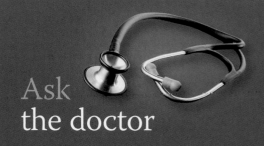

# Ask the doctor

ACCUTANE® HAS GOTTEN A LOT OF BAD PRESS. WHAT CAN I EXPECT?

The point is to decrease sebaceous gland activity and stop acne formation. If your skin doesn't feel dry, you need more! Your lips will be dry and you'll need constant lip balm. Your eyes may become dry, but usually that means we need to cut back on the dose. Your muscles may ache a little, especially if you're active. Elevated cholesterol levels are pretty common, too.

Babies conceived while on Accutane may have birth defects. The national iPledge system requires females of childbearing potential use two methods of birth control and take a monthly pregnancy test. You should not become pregnant while taking Accutane, or for one month after.

Now for the possible but uncommon side effects: Hair loss, which will return after you complete your course of Accutane. Also, it is possible to develop a low blood count or irritate your liver. To look out for this, you'll have a blood test every month.

Very rare side effects include a horrible headache—the worst of your life—which means you need to stop the medicine immediately and contact your doctor. There is a small chance that Accutane may increase the risk of depression. Close follow up is recommended, especially if you have a history of mood disorders.

Avoid laser procedures while on Accutane, and for six months after because of the increased risk of scarring.

# Acne treatments and how they work

| | |
|---|---|
| **Retinoids**<br>(RETIN A®, RETIN A MICRO®, DIFFERIN®, TAZORAC®) | Make skin turnover more regular. Decrease acne formation and diminishes fine wrinkles. |
| **Azelaic acid**<br>(AZELEX®, FINACEA™) | Decreases comedone formation. Lightens dark pigmentation. |
| **Benzoyl peroxide**<br>(BENZAC®, NEO-BENZ®, TRIAZ® PADS) | Decreases bacterial counts. When used with antibiotic, decreases development of bacterial resistance to that antibiotic. Also breaks up comedones. |
| **Salicylic acid**<br>(NEUTROGENA® OIL-FREE ACNE WASH, CLINIQUE ACNE SOLUTIONS, SALEX™) | Decreases bacterial counts, removes surface skin cells. Decreases comedone formation. |
| **Topical sulfur**<br>(KLARON® LOTION, PLEXION®, SULFACET®) | Decreases inflammation and bacterial counts |
| **Topical antibiotics**<br>(ERYTHROMYCIN, CLINDAMYCIN) | Decrease inflammation and bacterial counts |
| **Oral antibiotics**<br>(DOXYCYCLINE, MINOCYCLINE, TETRACYCLINE, BACTRIM™) | Decrease inflammation and bacterial counts |
| **Oral retinoids**<br>(ACCUTANE®) | Shrink sebaceous glands, normalize skin turnover |
| **Injectable steroids** | Decrease inflammation quickly |
| **Chemical peels and microdermabrasion** | Physically remove sticky skin cells and unblock pores. Reduce acne formation and make pores appear smaller. |
| **Oral contraceptives**<br>(ORTHO TRI-CYCLEN®, YASMIN®, YAZ®) | Lower androgen hormones that stimulate oil production |

# Megan's story

AGE: 28

CONCERN: ACNE AND ACNE SCARRING

TREATMENT: VBEAM
PERFECTA LASER AND SMOOTHBEAM
LASER FOR ACNE, FRAXEL
RE:STORE LASER FOR SCARRING

NUMBER OF TREATMENTS: 3

BEFORE

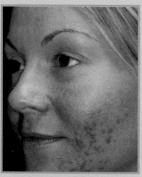

AFTER

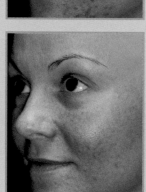

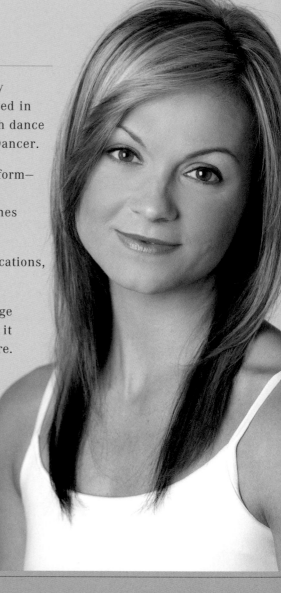

My passion is dancing and performing. It is my mode of artistically expressing myself, and I enjoy the bond with other dancers. I danced in college for the Texas State Strutters, and I've traveled the world with dance tours. I just completed my first year as a Houston Rockets Power Dancer.

When you are performing, appearance is crucial. My hair, body, uniform—and most importantly makeup—have to be flawless. I am constantly having my photo taken with fans and for print in calendars, magazines and posters. My job is to look good!

I suffered from acne throughout my teens and twenties. I tried medications, creams, ointments, glycolic peels, facials, and extractions.

Then I met a woman who was so passionate and open about the change laser treatment for acne had made in her life. After thinking about it for a day or so, I called to make an appointment for my first procedure.

The procedures were not very painful thanks to numbing cream, and there was no downtime after the VBeam and Smoothbeam lasers. After the Fraxel re:store, my face was red, a bit puffy and hot. But I applied ice packs and slept in an elevated position to prevent further swelling.

I felt great knowing my skin was healing from the inside out. I couldn't stop staring at myself in the mirror. It was amazing; my skin was so smooth and refreshed. After each procedure I could feel my skin getting smoother."

## PATIENT T!P

Seek a physician with a lot of experience treating acne, especially if you have darker skin. Treating an already inflamed area may lead to hyperpigmentation. A small amount of hyperpigmentation may be allowable and treated later with bleaching creams. Too much energy or cooling can lead to permanent hyperpigmentation and scarring.

# Acne scar solutions

Accutane is really a miracle for acne. But it does nothing to erase acne scars. Acne scars can be shallow "rolling" depressions or deep "ice-pick" crevices. Rolling scars respond the best to chemical peels and laser resurfacing. Reddish-brown flat dyspigmentation may also occur in the wake of acne. Dyspigmentation can be improved with bleaching creams, chemical peels, and lasers. Time usually improves redness. Enlarged pores are common in severe acne patients. Lasers can improve the appearance of acne scars and can reduce the size of pores.

The best thing for acne scars is prevention—please see your dermatologist early and don't hesitate to start the appropriate treatment, whether it's topical, oral antibiotics, or Accutane. If you already have scars, clear your acne, then seek a laser specialist to improve the scars. Technology is evolving every day, and each day our ability to address acne scars improves!

*Note: Wait at least six months after completing Accutane to start laser treatment.*

# What can we do about acne and acne scarring?

IN THE PAST FIVE YEARS, LASERS HAVE BEEN FOUND IN MULTIPLE STUDIES TO REDUCE NOT ONLY ACNE LESIONS BUT ALSO ACNE SCARS. Three popular laser systems for acne and acne scarring are the pulsed-dye laser, the 1450-nm diode laser, and fractionated lasers.

The pulsed-dye laser works by targeting blood vessels. Once the acne lesion is tampered with, chemical signals are sent out to recruit inflammatory cells to survey and clean up the area. Inflammatory cells come in via the blood vessels, squeeze out of the blood vessels, and surround the acne lesion. Lasers, such as the pulsed-dye laser, use heat to destroy blood vessels, eliminating the source of inflammation.

The 1450-nm diode laser is a longer wavelength so it penetrates deeper. It targets the sebaceous gland. Shrinking the sebaceous gland stops secretion into the follicle, stopping acne formation in its tracks. The long wavelength also heats collagen in the dermis, stimulating new collagen to form and fill in depressed scars.

Finally, fractionated photothermolysis systems like Fraxel heat columns of tissue. They can be adjusted to heat the dermis and stimulate collagen synthesis. The overlying epidermis is also heated, and with several treatment sessions, a resurfacing effect is achieved. This may unplug pores, improve depressed scars, and improve overall skin texture.

BEFORE

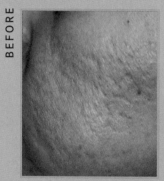

AFTER

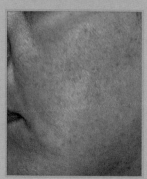

# Guide to acne and acne scarring treatments
## (what to expect with...)

| Treatment type | Brand options | Best for | Treatments | Cost |
|---|---|---|---|---|
| Pulsed-dye Laser | Candela® (Vbeam®, Vbeam® Perfecta) | Inflammatory acne vulgaris, rosacea, acne scarring | Feels like a rubber band snapping against your skin | $ |
| 1450-nm diode | Candela® (Smoothbeam®) | Acne, acne scarring, sebaceous hyperplasia | Requires 1-hour of topical anesthesia before treatment | $$ |
| Photodynamic Therapy | DUSA (Levulan® Kerastick® with blue light), Galderma® (Metvixia® with red light) | Acne | Topical photosensitizer is applied to the skin for 30-90 minutes followed by illumination with a laser or light source | $$ |
| Non-ablative Fractional Photothermolysis | Solta (Fraxel re:store™), Palomar (LUX 1540™), Cynosure® (Affirm™) | Acne scarring | Requires 1-hour of topical anesthesia before treatment | $$$ |
| Ablative Fractional Photothermolysis | Lumenis® (Ultra Pulse Active FX), Cutera® (Pearl™), Solta (Fraxel re:pair®), Palomar (LUX 2940™) | Acne scarring | Requires anesthesia (general, IV sedation, or blocks) | $$$$ |
| $CO_2$ and Erbium Resurfacing | Lumenis® (Coherent Ultrapulse), Derma-K®, Sharplan SilkTouch | Acne scarring | Requires anesthesia (general, IV sedation, or blocks) | $$$$ |
| Hyaluronic Acid Dermal Fillers | Restylane®, Perlane®, Juvéderm™ | Acne scarring | Topical anesthesia or dental blocks are optional, but may not be necessary depending on the patient. Feels like a needle prick. | Based on the amount of product used |

*Consult with your physician before discontinuing medication

| Recovery | Follow up visit | How it works | Tips |
|---|---|---|---|
| Bruising can last from 2 days to 2 weeks | 4–6 weeks, requires several treatments | Selective photothermolysis of the dilated vessels associated with inflammation | Avoid aspirin, vitamin E, caffeine, and alcohol 5 days before and after procedure* to reduce bruising. Apply ice to halt bruise formation. |
| Redness or swelling may develop, but patients return to work the same day | 4–6 weeks, requires several treatments | Shrinks oil glands and suppresses inflammation. Stimulates collagen production to improve acne scars. | Avoid sun exposure for 2 weeks before and after the laser procedure. |
| Mild peeling, redness and swelling for 2–4 days | 2–4 weeks, requires several treatments | Destroys acne-causing bacteria | Strict avoidance of sun exposure for 48 hours after the procedure is required. Even indoor lighting may cause redness and swelling. |
| Mild to moderate redness and swelling resolve within 48–72 hours | 4–6 weeks, requires several treatments | Stimulates new collagen formation and remodeling | Elevate area, ice frequently, and take anti-inflammatories or antihistamines to minimize swelling |
| Up to 2 weeks of moderate to severe inflammation, redness, and peeling | Close follow-up immediately following treatment | Partially removes the epidermis and dermis resulting in wound remodeling with subsequent new collagen and elastin formation | Expect 7–10 days of downtime |
| Up to 2 weeks of moderate to severe inflammation, redness, and peeling | Close follow-up immediately following treatment | Completely removing the epidermis and part of the dermis results in wound remodeling with subsequent new collagen and elastin fiber formation | Expect 7–10 days of downtime |
| Minor swelling and bruising for up to 7–10 days | Fillers last from 6 months up to a year. Will need touch-ups as results fade. | Act as temporary props making scars less noticeable | Icing after treatment will reduce inflammation and bruising |

| LEGEND | $ = $200–$500 | $$ = $501–$800 | $$$ = $801–$1100 | $$$$ = $1101 + |
|---|---|---|---|---|

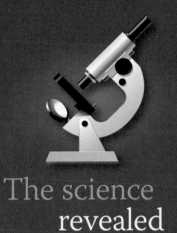

## The science revealed

THE 1450-NM DIODE WAS ONE OF THE FIRST LASERS REALLY SHOWN TO IMPROVE ACNE, AND EVEN ACNE SCARRING. The only problem is it can be a little painful. Each pulse is associated with a quick burst of pain, similar to a rubberband snapping against the skin. It takes about 100–200 pulses to cover the entire face, about 10 minutes. If you're worried about pain, treatment can be limited to your most stubborn areas. The good news is that as you have less acne, your skin is less inflamed and each pulse hurts less. Plus you can use topical numbing cream for 30–60 minutes before the treatment.

The laser seems to also decrease oiliness and acne scarring. You'll need about three monthly treatments, and results typically last 6–12 months. This is a great option for those who do not want to take Accutane.

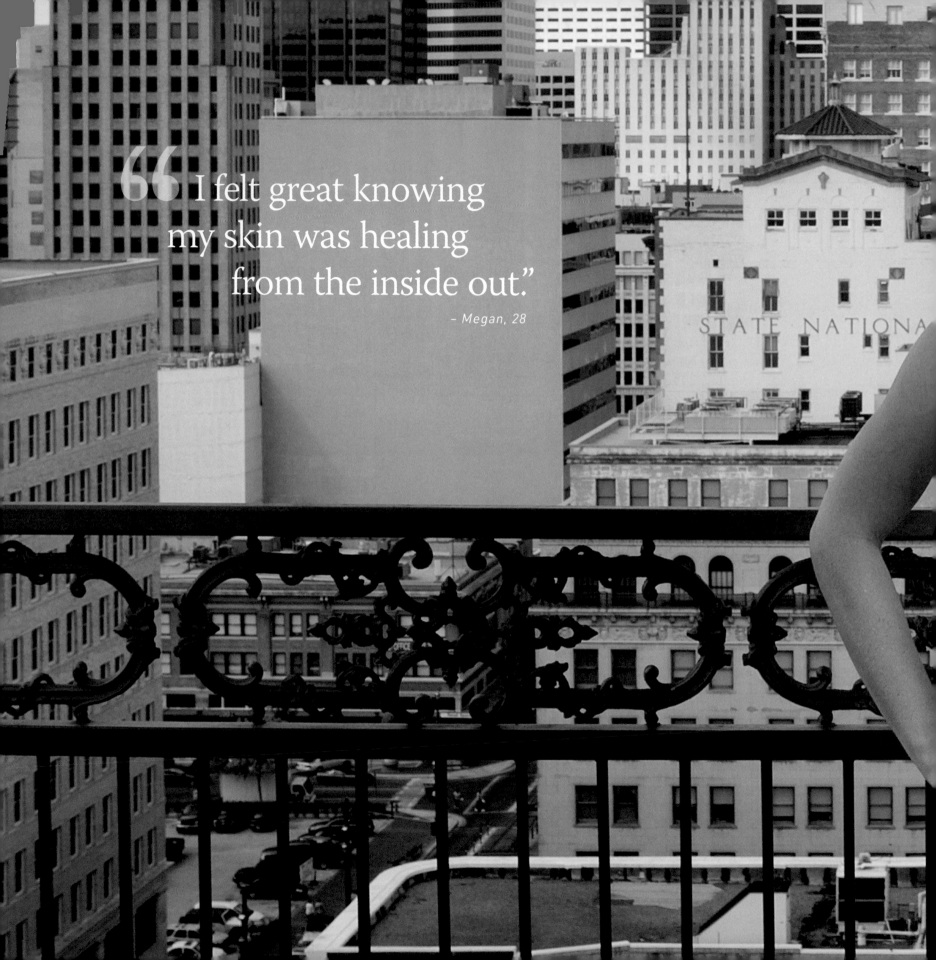

"I felt great knowing my skin was healing from the inside out."

– Megan, 28

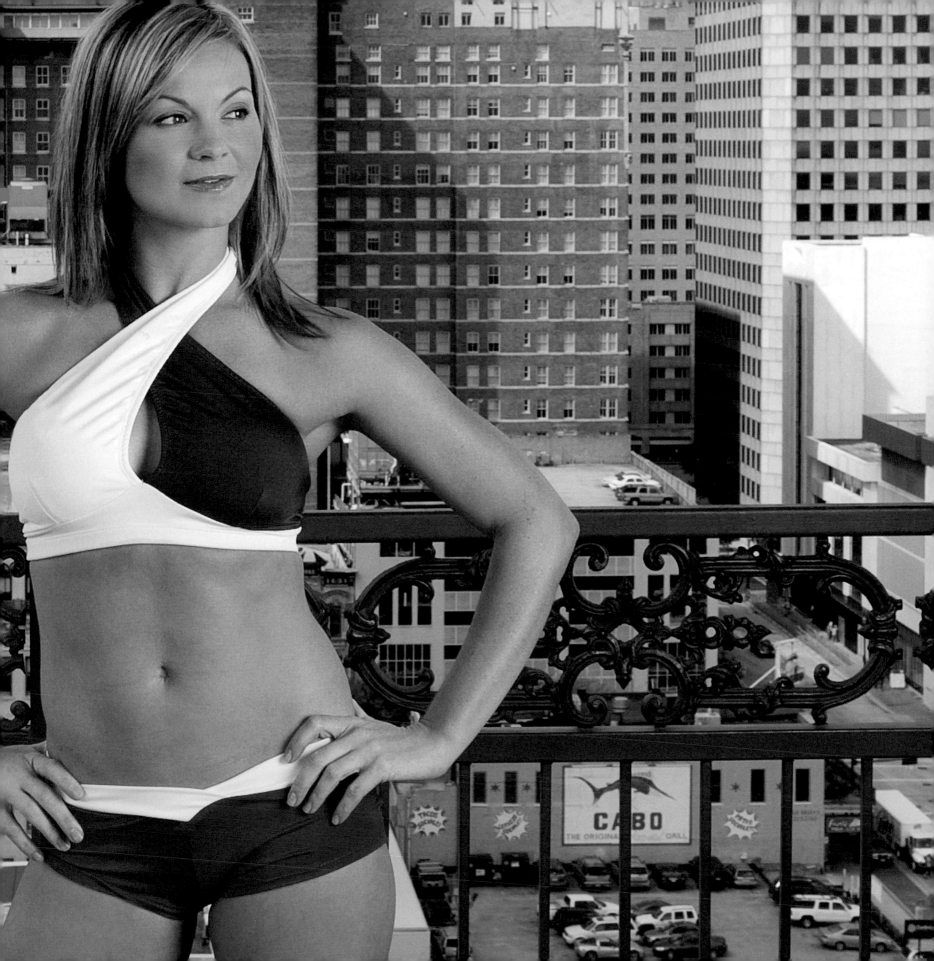

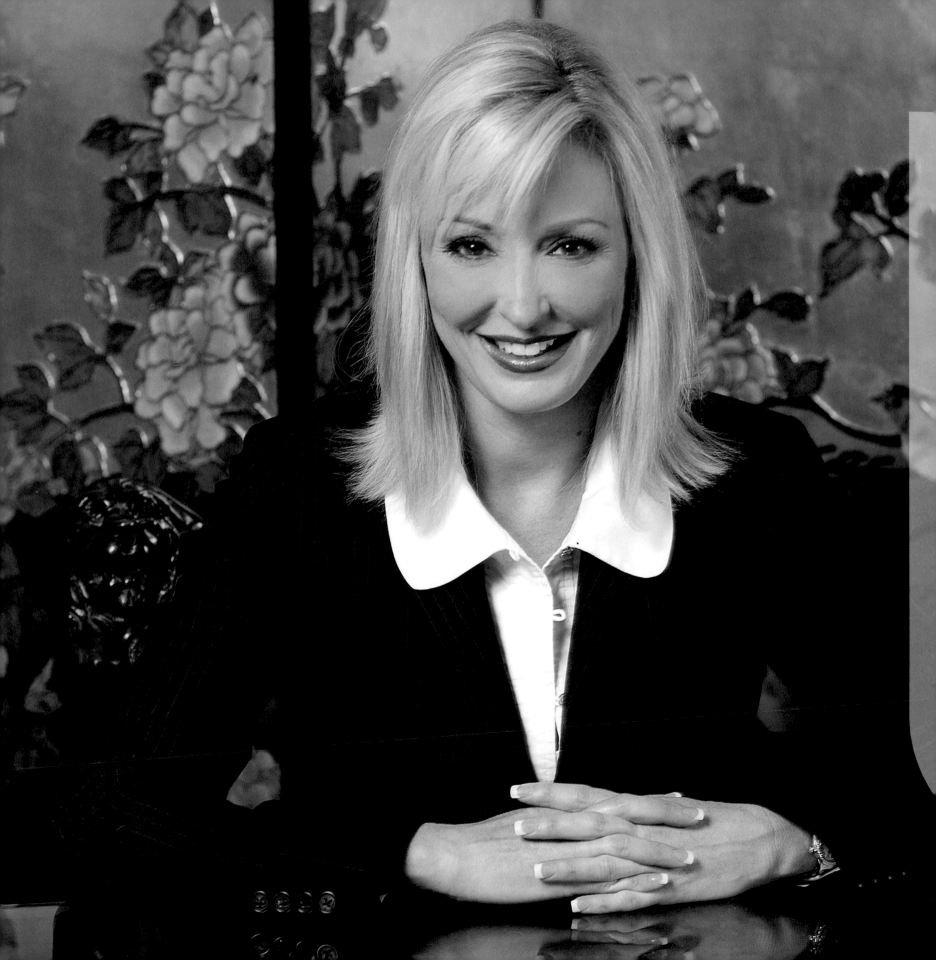

# WRINKLES

# CHAPTER 3

" **The appearance of fine lines**
        **on my thin lips**

CAUSED MY LIPSTICK TO BLEED INTO THE LINES."

– Vanessa, 50

Do you see fine, thin lines all over your face, or deep lines between your eyebrows and around your mouth? Are the lines there all the time, or only during certain facial expressions? The answers to these questions will guide your treatment choices. Reducing lines and hollows will project the appearance of youth and health.

# Why it occurs

FINE LINES AND TEXTURAL CHANGES ARE CAUSED BY SUN DAMAGE AND TIME. MANY YEARS OF SUN EXPOSURE DAMAGES THE ELASTIC FIBERS IMMEDIATELY BELOW THE SKIN'S SURFACE. With age, inflammatory chemicals break down supporting collagen. For smoothing and toning the skin, chemical peels, lasers, and light sources are recommended.

Fine lines, deeper wrinkles, and hollows are caused by time, facial expressions, and even how we sleep. Let's take a look at the two forms of aging:

1. **Wrinkles on the forehead and around the eyes:** Facial movements repeatedly crinkle the skin, creating wrinkles. This is most common around the forehead, between the brows, and around the eyes, because we use our brows and eyes to make expressions. Prominent brow muscles and the furrows between the brows eventually become permanent. This is a subconscious social cue, and one may be perceived as angry or negative by coworkers and friends.

2. **Hollows on the temples, under the cheekbones, and "parentheses" wrinkles framing the mouth:** We used to think that wrinkles were from gravity pulling down on loose skin, so the answer was facelifts that pulled the skin back and tucked it behind the ears. We've all seen pinched faces after bad facelifts; that's because even when the skin is tight, something is missing below the skin.

We now think most aging comes from volume loss. The skin is composed of elastic and collagen fibers swimming in a viscous matrix. With time, collagen is degraded and we make less matrix. The major substance in matrix is hyaluronic acid, a protein that absorbs water. Without collagen and matrix, the skin sags and areas of volume loss become apparent. Hollows form under the cheekbones on either side of the chin, causing skin to slide down and make jowls.

## PATIENT T!P

Reduce bruising by stopping aspirin, ibuprofen, vitamin E, herbal supplements, fish oil, and alcohol for one week prior to and after treatment. Please consult your physician before discontinuing medications.

# " Vanessa's story

The appearance of fine lines on my thin lips caused my lipstick to bleed into the lines. My doctor suggested filling the fine lines with Restylane. During my initial treatment for this condition, he also minimally augmented my lip line. I was thrilled with the results and my renewed ability to apply lipstick that remained intact all day. My lips are now beautifully full.

Botox and Restylane have erased my crow's-feet and nasolabial lines. I was in and out of the office in 30 minutes, with minimal bruising, and was able to go straight back to work.

My overall results have boosted my confidence tremendously. I look renewed.

I work in sales and believe looking younger has given me a leg up on those in the industry who are judged to be on the downward side of their career aspirations. My face can now match the energy and enthusiasm I have in my life."

AGE: 50
CONCERNS: AGING, SUN DAMAGE, FINE LINES
TREATMENT: BOTOX, RESTYLANE
DOWNTIME: NONE TO MINIMAL (24–48 HOURS)

BEFORE

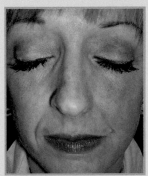

AFTER

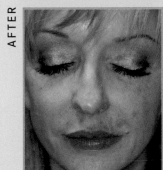

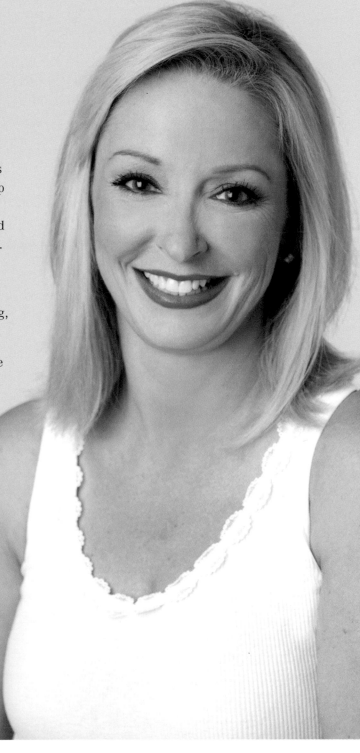

# Treatment options and how they work

THE TREATMENT FOR DYNAMIC WRINKLES RELAXES THE MUSCLES, WHILE THE TREATMENT FOR HOLLOWS AND RESULTING WRINKLES INVOLVES A DERMAL FILLER TO REPLACE VOLUME LOSS. For most people, a combination of techniques yields the best results. The best physicians are part artist, using multiple techniques and products to achieve your personal best.

Initially, these products were used only by the rich and famous. The unrealistic demand from Hollywood and inexperience of physicians led to overcorrection—frozen faces without expression and huge lips! Today's experienced physicians can create any amount of correction, from unnoticeable to very noticeable. The best will insist on creating a natural look so you can still raise your eyebrows, crinkle your nose, and smirk when appropriate.

**BOTOX® AND DYSPORT®** are purified forms of botulinum toxin. The only FDA-approved botulinum toxins for cosmetic use are medical grade Botox Cosmetic and Dysport.

Either Botox or Dysport is injected into the muscle and is taken up by the nerves that control that muscle. It makes the nerves unable to fire, so the muscle is not stimulated to contract. The effect lasts about four months.

Like any muscle not used, the treated muscle will become smaller, and perhaps down the road less medicine will be needed to achieve the same effect. If you have a really deep wrinkle, it will be greatly improved by Botox or Dysport, but it may take some time.

Generally, Botox and Dysport are used for wrinkles on the upper half of the face and the neck, which are mainly caused by muscle movement.

**FILLERS** Wrinkles on the lower half of the face tend to be a result of volume loss. Dermal fillers are injected beneath the wrinkle or hollowed area. The fillers most commonly used are made of hyaluronic acid, a substance that naturally occurs in the body.

**COLLAGEN FILLERS** were originally made from a cow source. Testing is done before treatment to make sure there is no allergic reaction. The Cosmoderm family of fillers is from a human source, so pre-testing is not necessary.

**RESTYLANE®** was the first available hyaluronic acid filler in the United States. It is made by Medicis, which also makes Perlane, a thicker version for deeper wrinkles. The product's effects last up to 18 months with one touch-up.

**JUVÉDERM™** is a hyaluronic acid filler made by Allergan (the company that produces Botox). Studies suggest it may last up to one year.

These products absorb water, which plumps up the skin, gives it volume, and softens overlying wrinkles. They may even stimulate new collagen formation.

**SCULPTRA™**, another popular filler, is a better choice for large areas of volume loss, particularly the hollows of the cheeks and temples. Filling under the cheekbone lifts the skin up away from the chin, reducing jowls. At least two, but probably three or four, monthly treatments are needed, and the correction will last up to two years.

**RADIESSE®** filler contains calcium-based microspheres suspended in a water-based gel. Once injected, this product stimulates the production of collagen to replenish lost facial volume. The effects may last 12 to 18 months.

**FAT TRANSFER** harvests fat (by liposuction of thigh, breast, neck, or other area) and injects it back into the same patient (to nasolabial folds, cheeks, temples, under the eyes, etc.). The harvested fat is kept in a refrigerator for up to a year so monthly treatments can be done. It often gives a natural, soft, but noticeable improvement that lasts months to years.

| Dermal filler | Where to use | Duration | Notes |
|---|---|---|---|
| Restylane® | Superficial wrinkles, nasolabial folds, lip augmentation, marionette lines | Up to 18 months with 1 touch-up | First hyaluronic acid filler to receive FDA approval in 2003 |
| Perlane® | Deeper wrinkles, nasolabial folds, marionette lines | About 6 months | May be used alone or in combination with Restylane |
| Juvéderm™ Ultra | Superficial wrinkles, nasolabial folds, lip augmentation, marionette lines | Up to 1 year | Contains the highest concentration of non-animal and cross-linked hyaluronic acid of any dermal filler currently available |
| Juvéderm™ Ultra Plus | Deeper wrinkles, nasolabial folds, marionette lines | Up to 1 year | Adds volume to the skin and may give the appearance of a smoother surface |
| Sculptra™ | Moderate to deep nasolabial folds, lipoatrophy | Up to 2 years | Restores and corrects the signs of facial fat loss |
| Radiesse® (CALCIUM HYDROXYLAPATITE MICROSPHERES) | Moderate to severe wrinkles and folds, lipoatrophy | 12–18 months | Can be mixed with lidocaine to minimize discomfort during injection |
| Zyderm® I (3.5% BOVINE COLLAGEN) | Superficial wrinkles, acne scars, lip augmentation | 3–5 months | 2 skin tests required 4 weeks apart |
| Zyderm® II (6.5% BOVINE COLLAGEN) | Moderate wrinkles | 3–5 months | 2 skin tests required 4 weeks apart |
| Zyplast® (3.5% CROSSLINKED BOVINE COLLAGEN) | Deeper wrinkles | 3–5 months | 2 skin tests required 4 weeks apart |
| Cosmoderm™ | Superficial wrinkles | 3–5 months | Skin testing not required before use. Virtually replaced Zyderm. |
| Cosmoplast™ | Deeper wrinkles | 3–5 months | Skin testing not required before use. Virtually replaced Zyderm. |
| Fat Transfer | Deep wrinkles and creases, plumping sunken/creased areas, lip/cheek augmentation | Can last just months or years, hard to predict | Requires several injection sessions for desired results |

# " Reba's story

In my 40s, I looked terrible due to the many wrinkles all over my face. I had cross-hatched lines everywherc and a deep line in my chin. I felt terrible about the way I looked. I tried tons of expensive products. I researched facelifts, mini facelifts, and other types of surgical procedures, but I was too nervous to try surgery.

After discussing my concerns with my dermatologist, we decided on the Fraxel re:store laser. Over the next five months, I endured monthly treatments. I say 'endured' because they were not pleasant.

However, I started seeing a difference in my face that made it all worthwhile. Even my husband noticed. The cross-hatched lines are almost entirely gone. My skin is much prettier. The deep line in my chin is no longer the focus of my face.

I look younger and don't feel like a grandmother (even though I am one)."

AGE: 54

CONCERN: PHOTOAGING

TREATMENT: FRAXEL RE:STORE

NUMBER OF TREATMENTS: 5

DOWNTIME: REDNESS & MINIMAL SWELLING FOR 3–4 DAYS

BEFORE

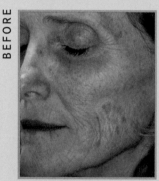

AFTER

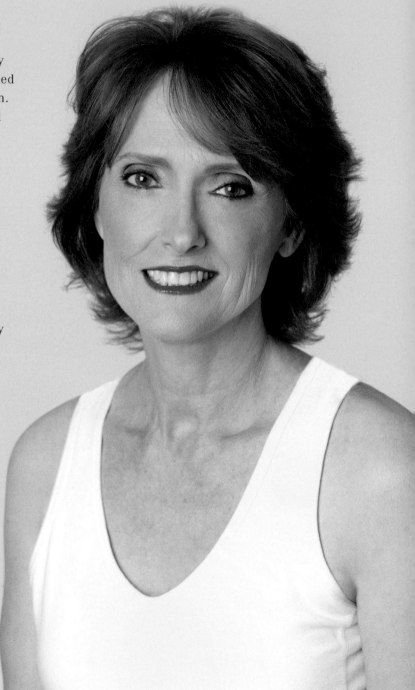

# What to expect
## (time, cost, recovery, permanence, risk)

**BOTOX® OR DYSPORT®** involves multiple tiny injections into the wrinkle area. The needle and amount of medicine injected is very small; each injection lasts less than a second. You'll feel pinpricks during the procedure. The tiny injection sites will heal in a few hours. This is truly a lunchtime procedure as you can go to work right away. Some experience a mild headache during the first 24 hours.

If you contract the muscle, 15 times every 15 minutes for the first one to two hours after treatment, your muscles may take up more of the medicine. This can result in an enhanced response. In three to five days improvement will be noted; however, the full effect will occur in one to two weeks.

All faces display subtle asymmetry. Either Botox or Dysport is used to correct this asymmetry as well as diminish wrinkles. More medication may be needed in some areas, while less is needed in others. If after two weeks you are uneven, return to your doctor for a touch-up. If you end up with an overcorrection, never fear—you'll look more natural in a month as the medicine is degraded.

The Botox effect should last four months. The fairest pricing is based on units used. If you have a big muscle, a deep wrinkle or a large area, the cost will be more. If you have a small wrinkle, it will be less. Some practices charge by the area. In that case, a forehead treatment will cost the same for a man with strong muscles or a petite woman with a single fine line. The other problem with pricing by the area is that you don't know how many units of medicine you are actually getting. The result will be the same, but won't last as long if too little product is used.

# What to expect
## (time, cost, recovery, permanence, risk) continued

**HYALURONIC ACID FILLERS** are usually injected in long lines under the skin. A larger volume of product is injected than with either Botox or Dysport, so the procedure can be a little more painful. Pre-treatment with topical anesthesia, injected anesthesia, or even a nerve block, like at the dentist, can be done based on preference. Hyaluronic acid fillers can be mixed with liquid anesthetic to minimize discomfort during injections. The good news: results are immediate!

Common side effects are swelling and bruising for up to one week, though many patients can go back to work immediately. Sometimes patients like the amount of correction received in part due to swelling, so a few days later, they feel that the product has worn off. Of course it hasn't, and more filler can always be added. On the other hand, if you think you received too much filler, change your mind, or the effect isn't smooth, there is an antidote. Hyaluronidase can be injected to break up the hyaluronic acid filler.

A rare complication occurs when the substance is injected into a blood vessel. The blood vessel becomes blocked and the overlying skin no longer receives blood, so it dies and becomes black like a scab. The more permanent the filler, the worse this complication can be. Often the area heals well, but scarring can occur.

**SCULPTRA™** is injected in long sweeping lines into large areas. The product is usually mixed with water and a liquid anesthetic. Anesthetic is delivered as the product is injected. The first few injections may be a little tender, but as the anesthetic takes effect, it usually becomes tolerable. Treatment around the sensitive mouth may still need a little pre-treatment numbing.

Results are not immediate. Patients are informed there will be NO improvement after the first treatment. Any volume improvement is due to swelling, and will be gone the next day. But over time as additional product is added, collagen synthesis occurs and the effect seen on the first day can be achieved. The first-day swelling is like a preview of what is possible with time.

The most common side effect is bruising, which can last up to two weeks. In clinical studies, about 3 percent of Sculptra patients developed tiny bumps around the injected product. The bumps can be felt by the patient but are rarely visible. Usually the nodules are tolerated, but sometimes they need to be cut out. A rare complication, as with all fillers, is accidental injection into a blood vessel.

**RADIESSE®** is injected in small amounts into the skin using a very fine needle. A topical anesthetic may be applied prior to treatment, or a liquid anesthetic may be mixed with the product to minimize discomfort. Results will be noted immediately. The product also stimulates collagen production so continued improvement will be seen over time. Common side effects are temporary swelling and bruising.

**FAT TRANSFER** involves harvesting of your own fat. Liposuction is performed to remove fat from behind your neck, on your abdomen, your thighs, or wherever you choose. A large liposuction procedure can be performed and some of the fat can be kept for use. Or, alternatively, a small liposuction procedure can be performed for the sole purpose of harvesting fat for transfer. After numbing the area, fat is removed with a wand placed under the skin. You'll feel pushing, pulling, and tugging as the wand is moved around under your skin. You may feel occasional twinges of pain if the wand comes into contact with a fibrous area.

The fat is then kept in syringes in a refrigerator. Each month, fat is injected into the desired site, such as the cheeks or under the eyes. The fat serves to fill in the area of volume loss, but can also stimulate new collagen formation. The duration of results is highly variable, and can last months or years.

Side effects include bruising and drainage at the liposuction site, and bruising at the recipient site.

A note on liposuction: Dermatologists and plastic surgeons are trained to perform liposuction. Tumescent anesthesia is an option during liposuction. This means the patient is awake and anesthesia is delivered via a long needle under the skin. Having the patient awake virtually eliminates the major risks of surgery: clots, death due to anesthesia, nausea after awaking from anesthesia, and heart and lung complications.

Liposuction involves passing a suctioning wand forward and backward under the skin. Liters of fat are removed so the result is seen immediately. However, as the skin heals and adheres back to the underlying fat and muscle, fibrous scarring occurs. This is actually what leads to most of the tightening, so the real result is not seen until 6 months, or even a year after the procedure.

**PATIENT T!P**

Avoid strenuous exercise, extensive sun or heat exposure, and alcoholic beverages for the first 24 hours following filler, Botox, or Dysport treatments.

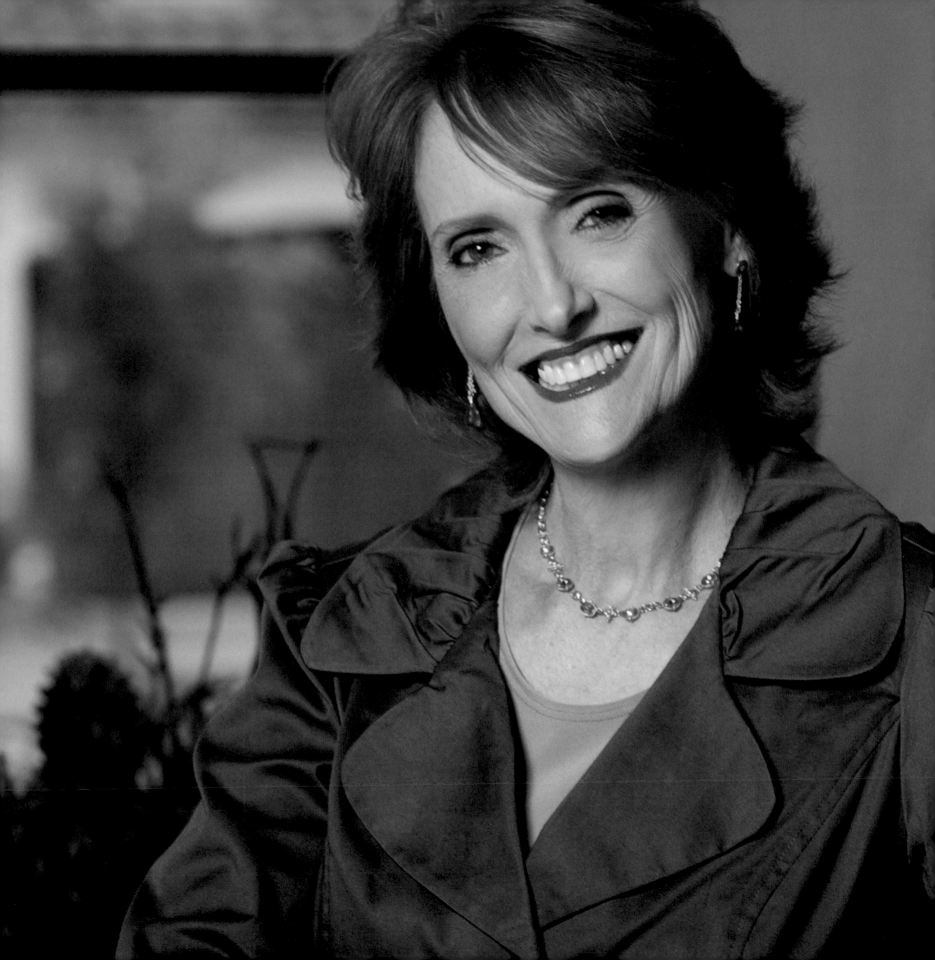

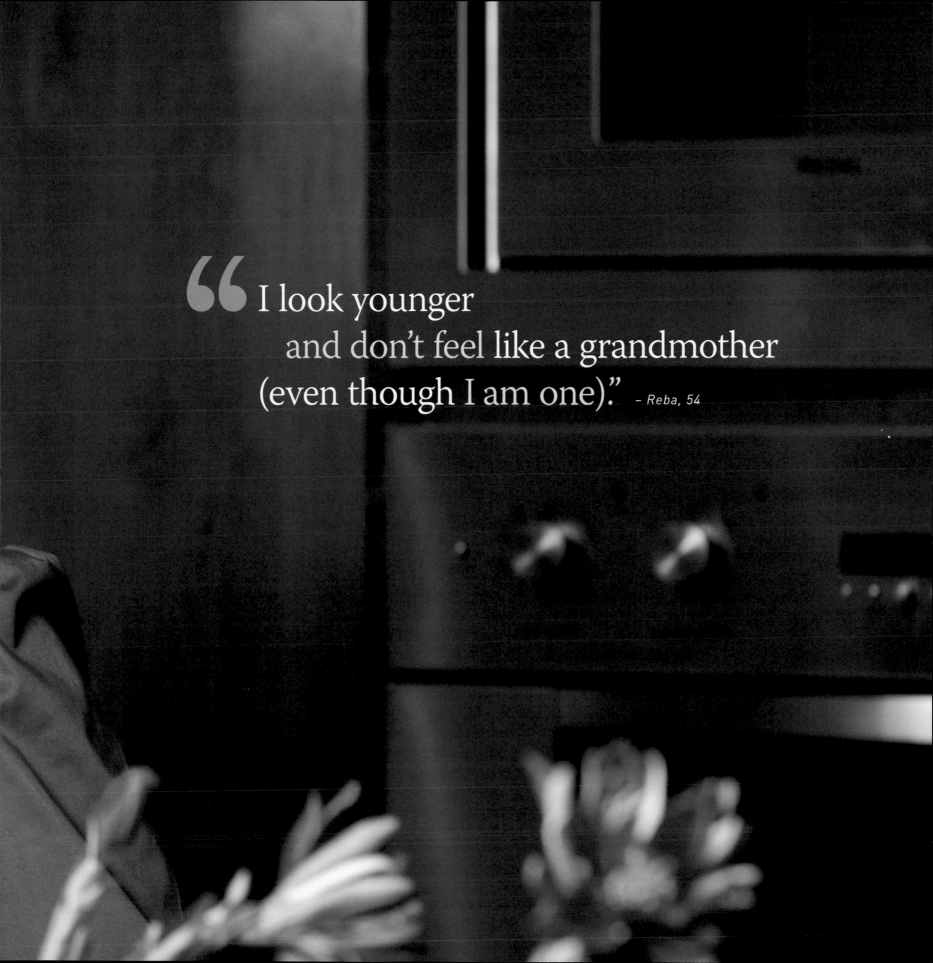

" I look younger and don't feel like a grandmother (even though I am one)." – *Reba, 54*

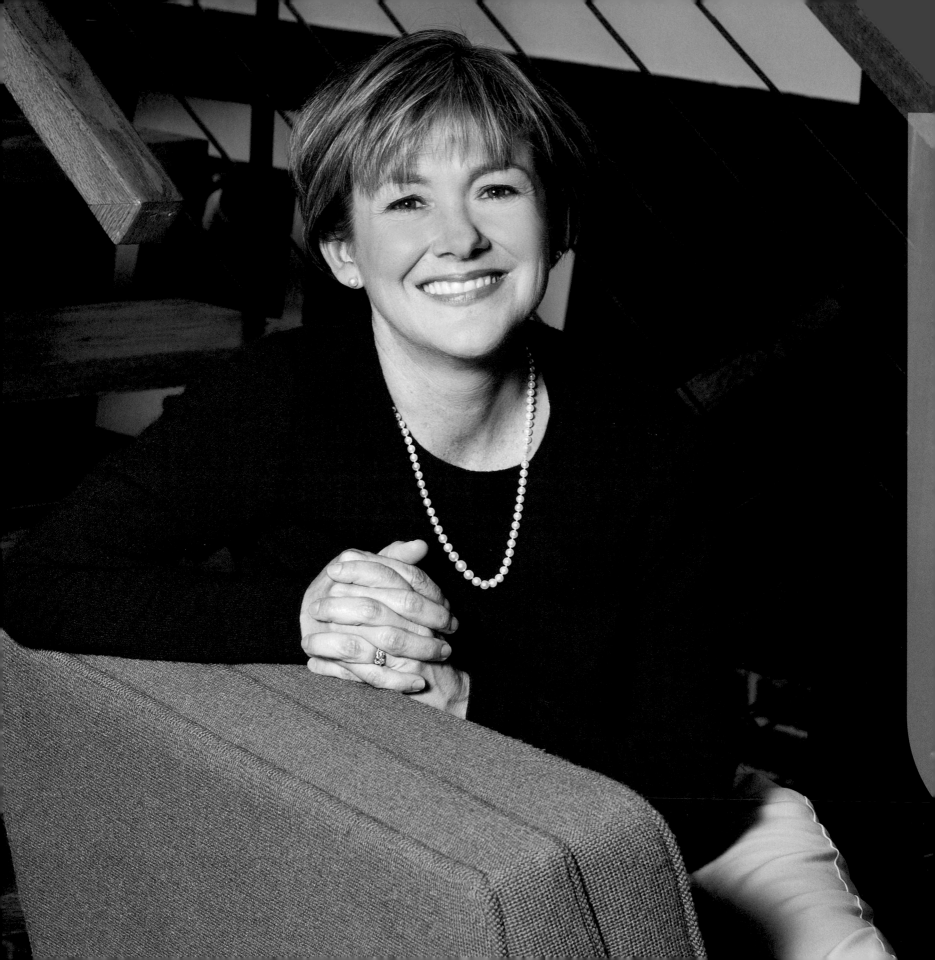

# RED ALL OVER

# CHAPTER 4

> " I teach elementary school and my students became so familiar with the afternoon flush that it was like a clock. AT AROUND 1:00 P.M. THEY WOULD ALL SHOUT OUT, 'THERE IT GOES. YOUR FACE IS REALLY, REALLY RED AGAIN.'"
>
> – Lyn, 43

Notable flushing, diffuse redness, and visible facial blood vessels all point to one of the most underdiagnosed, yet prevalent and frustrating skin conditions affecting adults. It is called rosacea. The symptoms vary considerably, each being responsive to a different course of treatment. The exact cause of rosacea is unknown, but dilated blood vessels and inflammation play a role. Common triggers to avoid and the treatments with the most promise are outlined in this chapter.

# Lyn's story

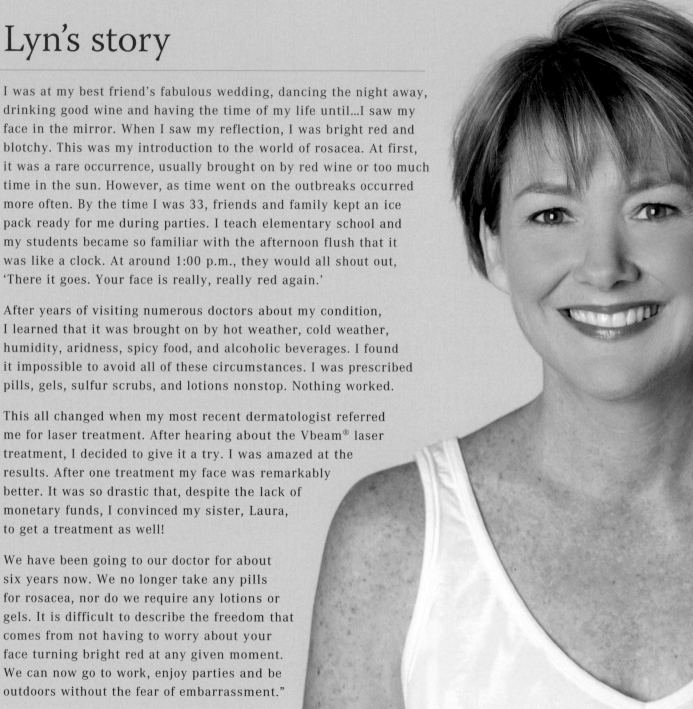

I was at my best friend's fabulous wedding, dancing the night away, drinking good wine and having the time of my life until...I saw my face in the mirror. When I saw my reflection, I was bright red and blotchy. This was my introduction to the world of rosacea. At first, it was a rare occurrence, usually brought on by red wine or too much time in the sun. However, as time went on the outbreaks occurred more often. By the time I was 33, friends and family kept an ice pack ready for me during parties. I teach elementary school and my students became so familiar with the afternoon flush that it was like a clock. At around 1:00 p.m., they would all shout out, 'There it goes. Your face is really, really red again.'

After years of visiting numerous doctors about my condition, I learned that it was brought on by hot weather, cold weather, humidity, aridness, spicy food, and alcoholic beverages. I found it impossible to avoid all of these circumstances. I was prescribed pills, gels, sulfur scrubs, and lotions nonstop. Nothing worked.

This all changed when my most recent dermatologist referred me for laser treatment. After hearing about the Vbeam® laser treatment, I decided to give it a try. I was amazed at the results. After one treatment my face was remarkably better. It was so drastic that, despite the lack of monetary funds, I convinced my sister, Laura, to get a treatment as well!

We have been going to our doctor for about six years now. We no longer take any pills for rosacea, nor do we require any lotions or gels. It is difficult to describe the freedom that comes from not having to worry about your face turning bright red at any given moment. We can now go to work, enjoy parties and be outdoors without the fear of embarrassment."

AGE: 43
CONCERN: ROSACEA
TREATMENT: VBEAM LASER
NUMBER OF TREATMENTS: 9
DOWNTIME: 2 DAYS

BEFORE

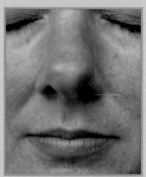

AFTER

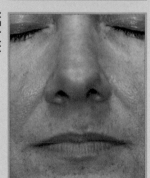

## What are the symptoms of rosacea?

You may have one symptom, or a combination of symptoms.

**THEY INCLUDE:**

**PERSISTENTLY RED NOSE AND CHEEKS**

**BURSTS OF REDNESS ON NOSE AND CHEEKS (flushing)**

**TINY, THREAD VEINS (telangiectases)**

**FACIAL SKIN SWELLING**

**ITCHING**

**BURNING**

**BUMPS THAT LOOK LIKE ACNE, BUT COME AND GO (papular rosacea)**

**PERSISTENT YELLOWISH BUMPS (sebaceous hyperplasia)**

**HISTORY OF STYES ON EYELIDS**

**EYES FEEL ITCHY, DRY, IRRITATED**

**EYES WATERY OR BLOODSHOT**

**OVERGROWTH OF NOSE**

## Why it occurs

IF YOUR FACE IS RED OR FLUSHED ON THE CHEEKS AND NOSE, YOU MAY HAVE ROSACEA. CLUES FOR ROSACEA ARE FLUSHING AND BURNING TRIGGERED BY HEAT, EXERCISE, AND RED WINE. There can also be small papules that look like acne. A tiny area composed of super-thin red or purple lines is a telangiectasia. These are simply dilated blood vessels. They may appear on the face as part of rosacea, or may appear on the face and elsewhere from trauma or sun damage. Rarely are telangiectases a sign of a more serious internal disease process.

Although the cause of rosacea is yet to be discovered, the leading theory maintains that increased blood vessels and vasodilation play a role. Chemicals leak out of the vessels and cause inflammation. New inflammatory molecules present in rosacea are being discovered every day. Both men and women can experience rosacea. Those with fair skin are particularly susceptible.

Another cause of redness is poikiloderma. This refers to red, brown, and white "spots" often occurring as the result of severe, long-term sun damage. Persistent bumpy and discolored skin can be seen on the sides of the neck and V of the chest. Spots, discolorations, and pigmentation are discussed in more detail in the chapters on complexion and general dermatology.

# Laura's story

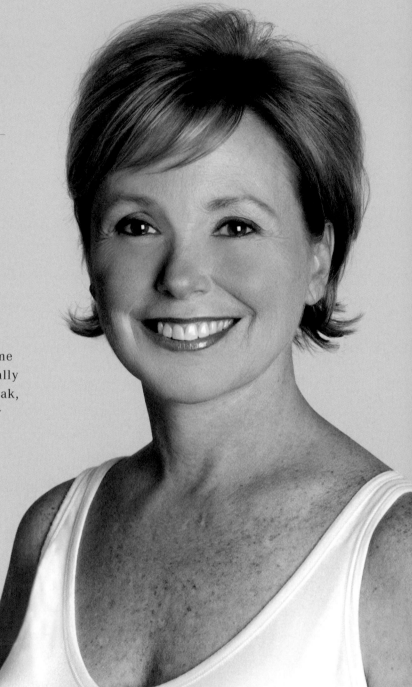

AGE: 49
CONCERN: ROSACEA
TREATMENT: VBEAM LASER
NUMBER OF TREATMENTS: 8
DOWNTIME: 2–3 DAYS OF
REDNESS & SWELLING WITH
OCCASIONAL BRUISING
FOR 5 DAYS.

**BEFORE**

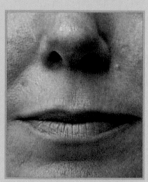

**AFTER**

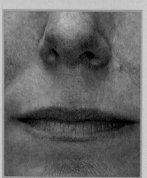

At 21 I first discovered I had rosacea. I was pregnant with my first daughter and my face started breaking out so badly that it actually hurt. I went to the dermatologist, not having any idea what I had. I thought it was just a symptom of pregnancy and that it would go away after I gave birth. I was shocked to hear I would always have rosacea.

Many times (especially when I got nervous), I could tell from people's expressions that I was turning red. I have even had people ask me if I am OK or if I need to sit down. I occasionally still get the feeling that I am having an outbreak, but when I check in the mirror there is barely any sign of redness.

This treatment has been the best thing ever for me. Without the laser treatments, I would have had to wear heavy makeup. I have recommended this treatment to everyone I know who suffers from rosacea. It has made a huge difference in my life."

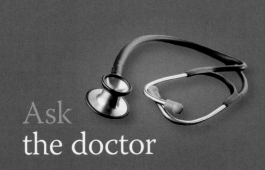

# Ask
# the doctor

## WHICH LASERS ARE USED TO TREAT ROSACEA?

The pulsed-dye laser targets broken blood vessels and background redness. It is important that patients realize that rosacea is a chronic condition, requiring periodic maintenance treatment after the initial series of treatments.

Adult acne, oily skin, and enlarged oil glands are also commonly associated with rosacea. These symptoms can be treated with the 1450-nm diode laser. Patients are able to undergo combination treatment with both lasers during the same office visit.

In general it is safer not to treat tanned skin with this laser technology, so patients should take precautions to avoid excess sun exposure both before and after their treatment sessions.

# Treatment options

SINCE ROSACEA IS DUE TO VASODILATION AND INFLAMMATION, IT CAN SOMETIMES BE ADEQUATELY CONTROLLED WITH TOPICAL MEDICATIONS AND ORAL ANTIBIOTICS. Still, redness may persist, making patients flush and appear nervous or sunburned. In this case, the vascular component can be treated with the pulsed-dye laser, which targets red blood cells. The surrounding blood vessel is heated and collapses. If the blood vessel bursts, a few blood cells leak out, creating a temporary bruise.

The laser is used to treat the entire affected area, whether evident on the nose, cheeks, or forehead. Three to five monthly treatments should make a big difference, with typically 50 percent to 75 percent improvement. Maintenance treatments are performed at three to six month intervals.

The pulsed-dye laser can also be used for small facial blood vessels unrelated to rosacea. The laser beam can be focused exclusively on the dilated vessel. One or two pulses may be all that are necessary. The blood vessels may refill and need one or two additional treatments to completely close. An alternate treatment is heating the vessel with a fine needle.

For poikiloderma mainly made up of telangiectases (tiny blood vessels), the pulsed-dye laser is applied to the entire affected area. Three to five monthly treatments may be needed. Other treatment options for poikiloderma include intense pulsed light (photofacial) and fractional laser treatment.

# What to expect
## (time, cost, recovery, permanence, risk)

THE PULSED-DYE LASER HAS A COOLING MECHANISM BUILT INTO THE LASER HAND PIECE. Every time the physician pulls the trigger, the laser emits a cooling spray milliseconds before emitting the laser light. The cooling spray condenses when it hits the skin, causing the surface of the skin to be cooled and protected from laser light. This way only the underlying vascular structures are heated. Cooling also mediates pain, so topical anesthesia is not always necessary. In fact, anesthesia may constrict blood vessels, eliminating the target and reducing effectiveness.

What will you feel? Because of this built-in cooling spray, you'll likely feel a quick burst of energy (like a rubber band snapping against your skin) with a burst of cool air (like someone blowing air on you). Even through protective eyewear, you will see a bright flash of light. The sensation of rubber band snapping, cool air, and bright light lasts less than one second and occurs with every pulse.

The number of pulses needed depends on the size of the treatment area. Slightly overlapping pulses are placed in an orderly fashion up and down the cheeks. Similar pulses are used to treat the entire neck and chest for poikiloderma. In contrast, only a couple of pulses are needed to treat a telangiectasia or angioma. The treatment of congenital and infantile vascular lesions is complex and varies from patient to patient (See Chapter 5).

Cost will depend on how many pulses are used. Some practices charge by the area, i.e. the face, the neck, or the lesion. Other practices charge by the pulse. In general, one full face session may cost about $500. A single lesion may be treated for about $250. Again, multiple treatment sessions are usually needed.

Rosacea responds very well to laser treatment. Patients tired of using creams or remembering to take a pill every day appreciate the lasting results seen with laser treatment. Keep in mind the laser targets the vessels, but does not stop the rosacea process. Rosacea is never completely cured; therefore the redness and/or bumps may slowly come back, making annual maintenance treatments necessary.

Poikiloderma has variable results depending upon the color of the spots. Pulsed-dye laser only treats the red spots, so brown spots and a bumpy texture will not be improved. If the brown splotches and bumps are what bother you the most, a different treatment modality such as a fractionated non-ablative laser may be better for your particular condition.

Both telangiectases and angiomas are very amenable to treatment. Superficial and tiny telangiectases should completely resolve after one or two treatments. Results with congenital and infantile vascular lesions vary, and the goal may not be complete resolution but just significant lightening (See Chapter 5).

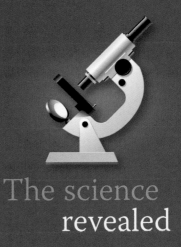

## The science revealed

THE PULSED-DYE LASER WAS INVENTED IN THE EARLY 1980s TO TREAT VASCULAR BIRTHMARKS. THE LATEST PULSED-DYE LASER TECHNOLOGY CAN BE SAFELY USED TO IMPROVE A NUMBER OF DIFFERENT CONDITIONS, SUCH AS ROSACEA, POIKILODERMA, RED SCARS, RED STRETCH MARKS, LEG VEINS, AND EVEN WARTS. Bruising was a common side effect of the original pulsed-dye laser, but the newer devices have longer pulse durations which minimize this potential side effect. After consulting with your physician, the discontinuation of aspirin, ibuprofen, Vitamin E, herbal supplements, and alcohol seven to 10 days prior to your treatment may also reduce the risk of bruising.

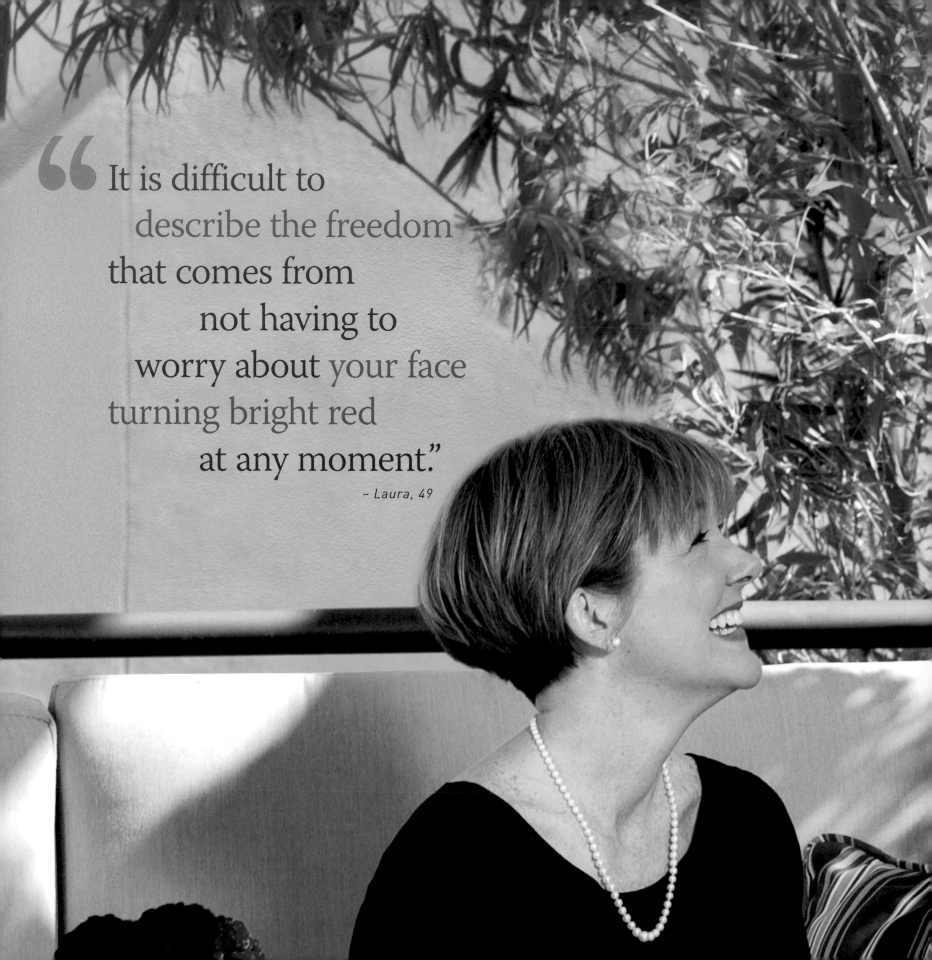

"It is difficult to describe the freedom that comes from not having to worry about your face turning bright red at any moment."

*– Laura, 49*

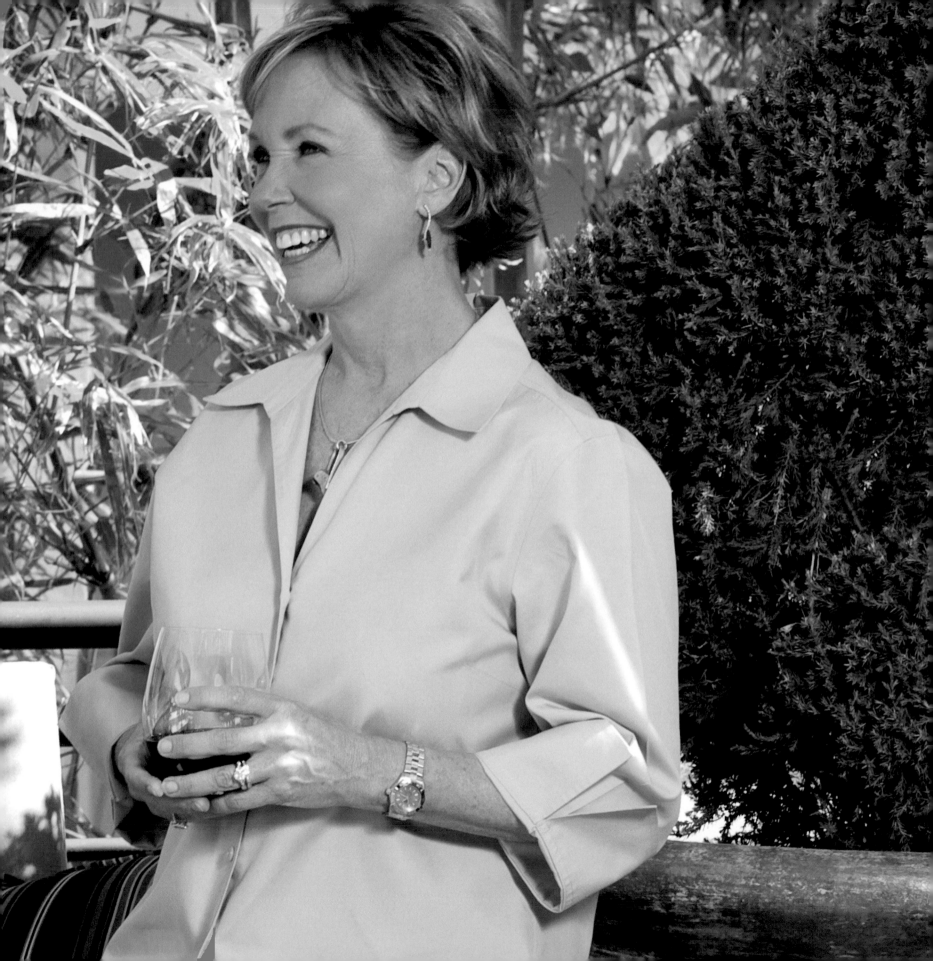

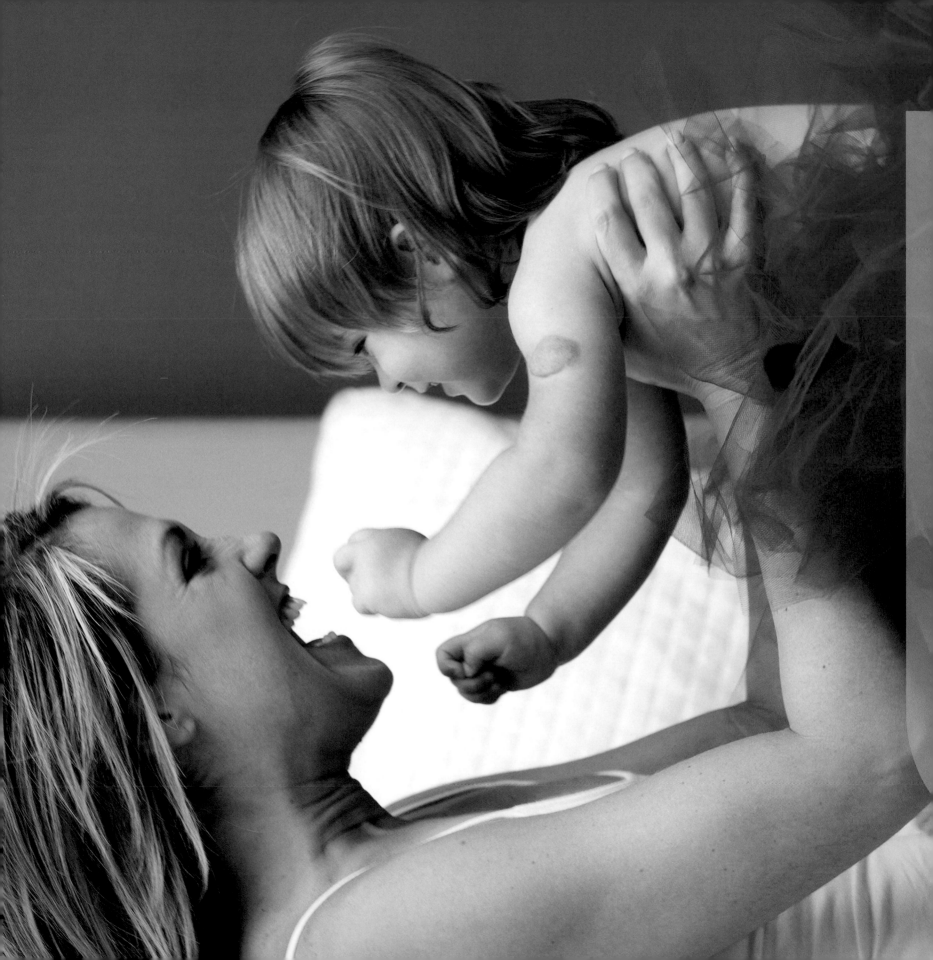

# BIRTHMARKS

# CHAPTER 5

> **I began to think I would have this mark on my face** FOR THE REST OF MY LIFE."
>
> *– Tara, 35*

Birthmarks may be present at birth or develop within the first few weeks of life. They can be brown, tan, blue, pink, or red. The most common birthmarks will be reviewed here: pigmented birthmarks and vascular birthmarks. A board-certified dermatologist, pediatrician, or facial plastic surgeon can determine the type of birthmark you have and the correct treatment. Lasers can be successfully used to treat a variety of birthmarks. Even some of the most complex birthmarks can now be treated with minimal risk of scarring.

# " Tara's story

It wasn't until after the fact that I realized how much my birthmark affected me and distracted others. I have had a pea-sized light brown birthmark on my left cheek for as long as I can remember. As a temporary solution, my dermatologist performed several in-office procedures where she used a 'freezing' technique directly on my birthmark.

The color lightened and faded, but because it was so textured, my skin in that area had a different look and feel than the rest of my face. During my first pregnancy, my birthmark became more pronounced, getting darker and more textured.

I was told surgery was not an option because the scar would be far worse than the original birthmark but was assured laser treatment could eliminate both the discoloration and textural differences to match the rest of my face. It took only two treatments and the birthmark completely went away. It was painless and provided the results I had given up hope of ever achieving.

Looking at my pictures now versus even a year ago, the difference is tremendous. It's a great example of a relatively minor procedure having a huge impact on the way I feel about myself and the impression I give others."

AGE: 35
CONCERN: BROWN BIRTHMARK
TREATMENT: ERBIUM:YAG LASER
NUMBER OF TREATMENTS: 2
DOWNTIME: 1 WEEK

BEFORE

AFTER

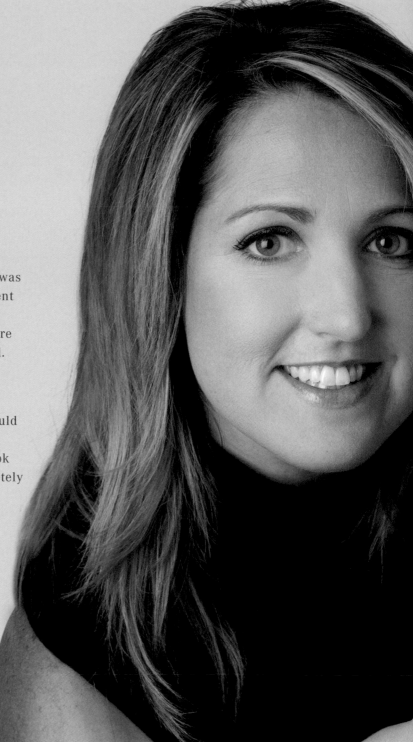

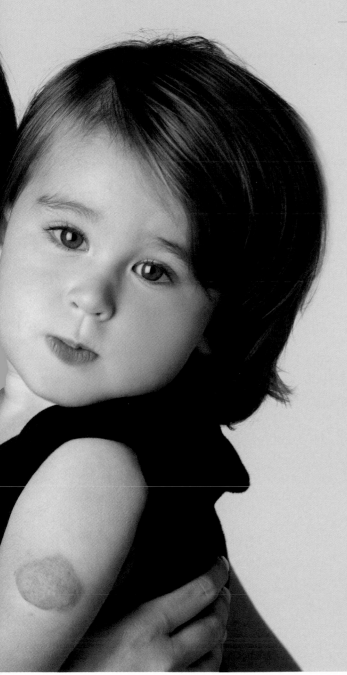

 # Manning's story

My daughter, Manning, was born with a small pink birthmark on her upper left arm that grew into a very large, thick, blood-red birthmark by the time she was a few months old. We learned from her pediatrician that her birthmark was called a hemangioma. Although it was not a health risk, and we were informed that it would most likely resolve by age 10, we wanted to understand everything we could about her birthmark and were referred to a specialist.

I had great luck with the lasering of my own birthmark and trusted the doctor who performed the procedure completely, so I had him look at Manning to see if something could be done for her as well. On her first visit, he assured me her hemangioma could be safely treated with laser technology, which would slow the growth process of her birthmark. She had nine monthly treatments that have significantly decreased the size and minimized the blood-red color of the hemangioma.

It is almost flat now and is nearly the color of her skin. While Manning doesn't always love the treatments, the professional staff are beyond kind to her and my family. They treat her so well that it makes me feel assured that I did the right thing for Manning and her birthmark."

AGE: 2
CONCERN: HEMANGIOMA
TREATMENT: VBEAM LASER
NUMBER OF TREATMENTS: 7
DOWNTIME: 1 WEEK

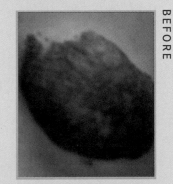

BEFORE

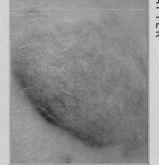

AFTER

## Why birthmarks occur

WHILE THE EXACT CAUSE IS UNKNOWN, WE DO KNOW THAT HEREDITY AND SPECIFIC ACTIVITIES DURING PREGNANCY HAVE NOTHING TO DO WITH A BABY DEVELOPING A BIRTHMARK. It is likely the result of an error during the formation of blood vessels or pigment when the baby is growing in the uterus. While in the womb, skin cells migrate from an area near the spinal cord around the sides and toward the front of the body. Pigment cells follow the same route. If one pigment cell gets confused and stops along that path, then a dark streak or patch results.

# Brown birthmarks, red birthmarks, and hemangiomas

**"CAFÉ AU LAIT"** is French for "coffee with milk." Café au lait spots are small or palm-sized flat areas of skin with a milky brown or light tan color. The patch ends abruptly so there is a clear distinction between the patch and surrounding skin. This is a common birthmark and almost always benign. However, having several of these marks can signal a rare genetic disorder and should be examined by a physician.

**NEVUS OF OTA** is a gray-brown patch around the eye, most common in Asians. Sometimes pigmentation of the eye accompanies this lesion. Rarely, melanoma, glaucoma, and neurological problems occur. Nevus of Ito is a similar gray-brown patch on the shoulder. These can appear at birth, shortly after birth, or during adolescence. Because the pigment cells are located deeper in this type of lesion, the brown patch can have a gray or blue tinge.

**CONGENITAL MOLES** look like regular moles, but are present at birth. They may be slightly larger and darker. The most common form is a thumb-print sized dark brown flat or raised area. Hair may grow out of the moles. These are benign. The risk for developing a melanoma within a congenital mole is similar to that of a regular mole (that develops during childhood or adolescence). Only congenital moles larger than 20 cm in diameter have a higher risk for developing melanoma, about 6 percent.

**CAPILLARY MALFORMATIONS** are usually present at birth. These generally do not enlarge, though they do "grow" proportionately with the infant. Faint red or purplish patches are commonly called "stork bites" or "salmon patches" when seen on the back of the neck. It can become darker red with exertion, such as when a baby cries or an adult exercises. Most of these capillary malformations are benign and do not require treatment.

**PORT WINE STAINS** are a type of capillary vascular malformation. They are red or purple areas that can occur anywhere, but often on the face. These are darker than stork bites, and can be thicker or slightly bumpy. They do not resolve on their own, and in fact, they usually grow deeper and thicker with time, making treatment more difficult. It is best to initiate laser treatment early on, as early as three weeks old. A physician should make sure there are no associated brain or eye abnormalities.

One in 10 babies develops a small **INFANTILE HEMANGIOMA** in the first few months of life. It begins as a red or purple bump that rapidly enlarges often causing alarm. After several months the lesion stops growing. Over the next few years the lesion turns dusky purple and resolves on its own. Generally, these are benign and do not need treatment; however they can sometimes leave permanent scars.

A dermatologist or pediatric dermatologist should make sure there are no associated problems and evaluate infantile hemangiomas. Infantile hemangiomas on the face or near important structures like the eyes need medical and sometimes laser or surgical treatment. A more complete overview of infantile hemangiomas can be found at www.birthmarks.com.

There are other vascular birthmarks, such as rapidly involuting congenital hemangioma, non-involuting congenital hemangioma, venous malformation, and arteriovenous malformation (AVM). These are rare and need to be evaluated immediately.

A cluster of overgrown blood vessels that makes a small bluish-red or cherry-red bump is an **ANGIOMA**. It is also called a "cherry angioma." Most people start noticing these cherry-red bumps around age 30-40, or sooner if they have fair skin. This type of hemangioma should not be confused with an infantile hemangioma.

## Michael's story

Many doctors have treated me over the last 10 years for my birthmark. My criteria are quite demanding in regard to the doctor, the equipment, staff, and quality of the treatment. Being in the hands of a capable laser surgeon provides me great peace of mind.

I spend time working on various entrepreneurial startups, tickling my youngest daughter, and fretting about my teenage daughter. I cherish my lovely wife, ride mountain bikes, and struggle with yoga. I try to appreciate the blessings in my life every day: my health, family, and friends. I can do all this with peace of mind knowing my birthmark has improved and wish this for others with birthmarks too. That's why I created www.birthmarks.com."

AGE: 49
CONCERN: PORT WINE STAIN
TREATMENT: VBEAM LASER
NUMBER OF TREATMENTS: 15
DOWNTIME: 7–10 DAYS
SWELLING AND BRUISING

BEFORE

AFTER

# "Karen's story

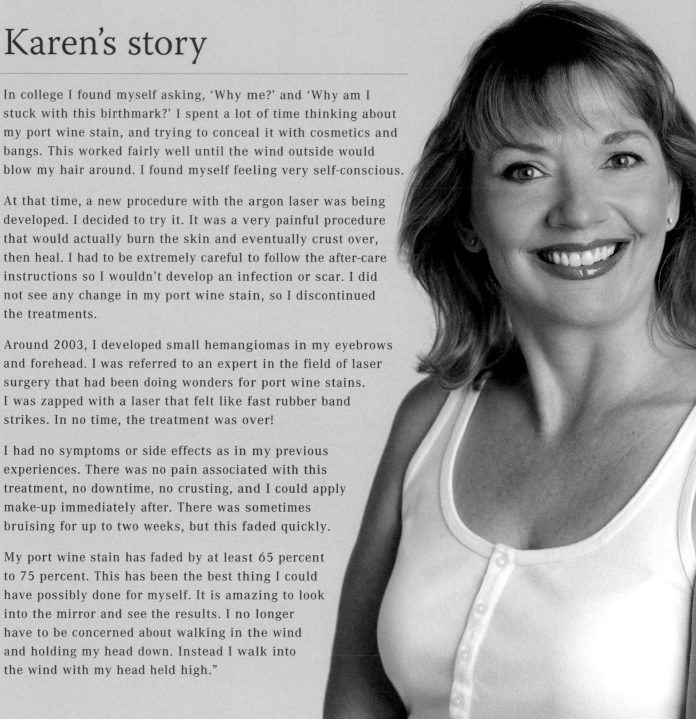

In college I found myself asking, 'Why me?' and 'Why am I stuck with this birthmark?' I spent a lot of time thinking about my port wine stain, and trying to conceal it with cosmetics and bangs. This worked fairly well until the wind outside would blow my hair around. I found myself feeling very self-conscious.

At that time, a new procedure with the argon laser was being developed. I decided to try it. It was a very painful procedure that would actually burn the skin and eventually crust over, then heal. I had to be extremely careful to follow the after-care instructions so I wouldn't develop an infection or scar. I did not see any change in my port wine stain, so I discontinued the treatments.

Around 2003, I developed small hemangiomas in my eyebrows and forehead. I was referred to an expert in the field of laser surgery that had been doing wonders for port wine stains. I was zapped with a laser that felt like fast rubber band strikes. In no time, the treatment was over!

I had no symptoms or side effects as in my previous experiences. There was no pain associated with this treatment, no downtime, no crusting, and I could apply make-up immediately after. There was sometimes bruising for up to two weeks, but this faded quickly.

My port wine stain has faded by at least 65 percent to 75 percent. This has been the best thing I could have possibly done for myself. It is amazing to look into the mirror and see the results. I no longer have to be concerned about walking in the wind and holding my head down. Instead I walk into the wind with my head held high."

**AGE: 45**
**CONCERN: PORT WINE STAIN**
**TREATMENT: VBEAM LASER**
**NUMBER OF TREATMENTS: 10**
**DOWNTIME: 5–7 DAYS**
**BRUISING**

BEFORE

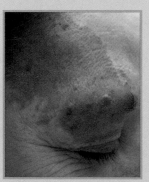

AFTER

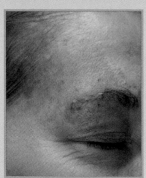

# Treatment and risks

**TREATMENT OF PIGMENTED BIRTHMARKS**: To reiterate, café au lait patches and congenital moles are benign but should be evaluated by a dermatologist. Small lesions can be surgically excised. Larger lesions can be treated with a laser that targets pigment, such as the Q-switched Nd:YAG, alexandrite, or ruby laser.

**TREATMENT OF VASCULAR BIRTHMARKS**: KTP and pulsed-dye lasers target vascular lesions. The laser emits light which is selectively absorbed by blood vessels, heating them and causing them to collapse.

If the vessel is heated and breaks open, red blood cells can leak out and a bruise will appear. There is typically bruising following each treatment session that will last approximately seven to 14 days. Avoiding medications and vitamins that thin the blood can help reduce the risk of bruising, as can the application of ice for 15 minutes after treatment. Though bruised, your skin should be intact and you can go back to work immediately after treatment. Settings can be adjusted to minimize bruising, but this usually means the treatment will be less effective. You may prefer shorter downtimes and be willing to undergo more treatments; just let your doctor know.

Any laser treatment in patients with dark skin can lead to hypopigmentation or hyperpigmentation. Seek a physician who has experience treating dark-skinned patients. The type of laser, amount of energy, and cooling settings can be adjusted to decrease the risk for dyspigmentation. Sometimes bleaching agents may be used before or after treatment to prevent or correct hyperpigmentation.

Other side effects are blistering and scarring. Carefully choosing effective but safe settings will help avoid permanent scars.

During the treatment, the eyes will be protected with appropriate eye protection. Infants less than 2 years old often tolerate the procedure if they are held by their parents. As the child becomes older and stronger, sedation in a controlled hospital setting may be used.

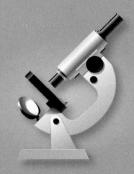

## The science revealed

PATIENTS MAY SEE UP TO 75 PERCENT TO 80 PERCENT IMPROVEMENT IN THE APPEARANCE OF THEIR PORT WINE STAIN BIRTHMARK FOLLOWING A SERIES OF PULSED-DYE LASER TREATMENTS. Alternatively, the pulsed-dye laser combined with the 1064-nm Nd:YAG laser, called the Cynergy™ laser, uses two wavelengths synergistically to treat port wine stains. However, with earlier intervention during infancy more patients may achieve complete clearing. Recent studies have shown that port wine stain clearance may be hastened by initiating treatment as young as 3 weeks of age.

The risks from these laser treatments are small. Textural and pigmentary irregularities following treatment are rare. The level of success in the treatment varies based upon the anatomical location and thickness of the port wine stain.

"I no longer have to be concerned about walking in the wind and holding my head down."

– Karen, 45

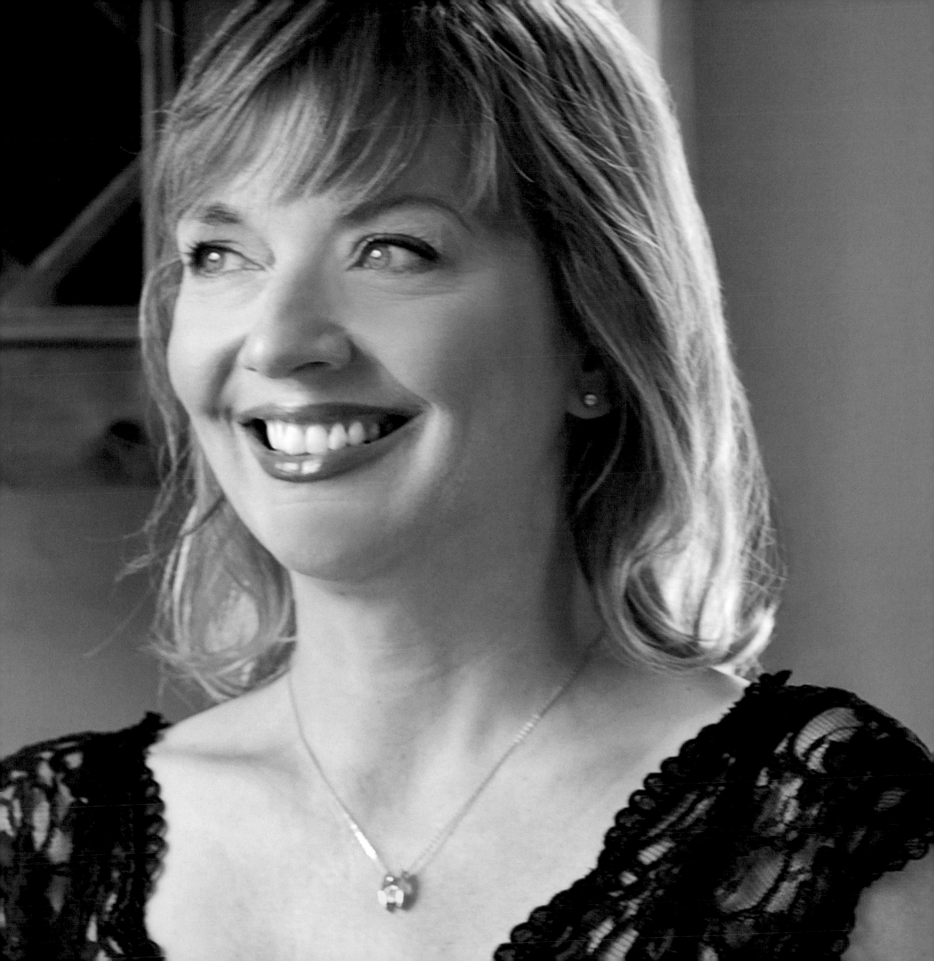

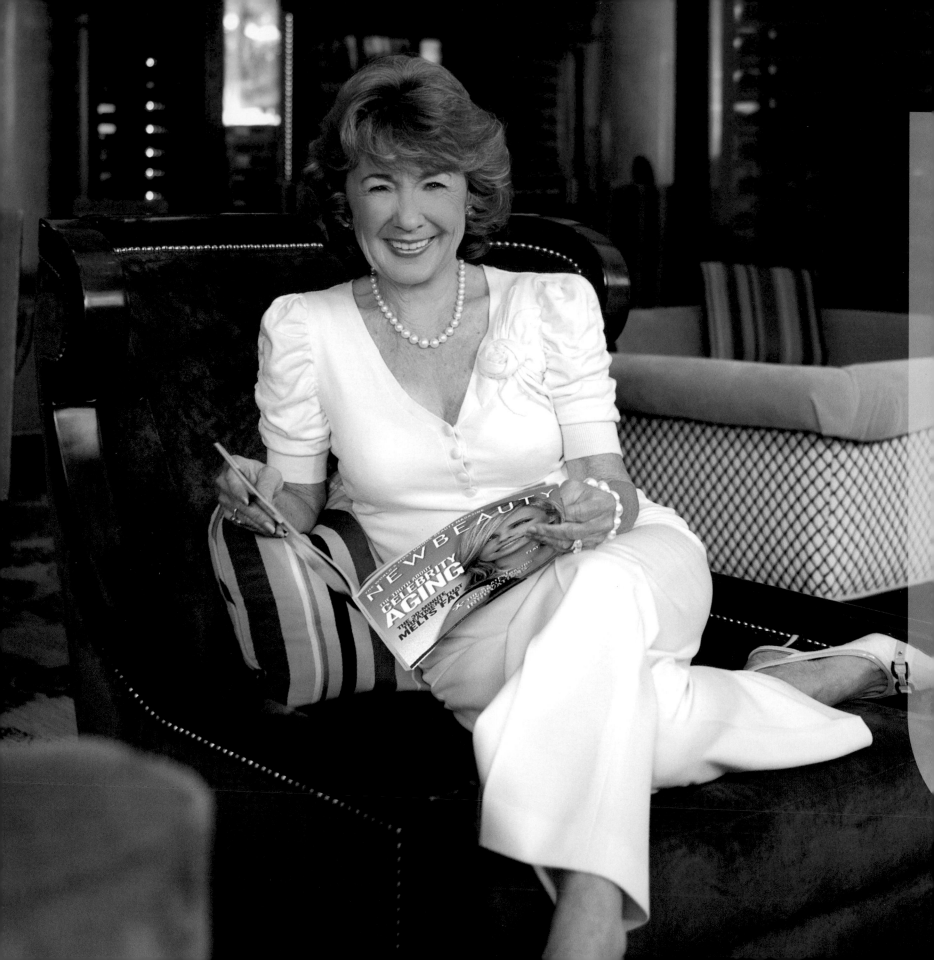

# EYES

# CHAPTER 6

" Losing my husband five years ago in an accident caused great stress,

**WHICH SHOWED UP IN MY FACE."**

*– Fran, 71*

Research shows we are constantly evaluating facial expressions for context. In a conversation your every facial move is subconsciously evaluated and interpreted. Your eyebrow arching upward may be perceived as surprise; the creases at the edge of your eyes may crinkle and give away your disapproval. Truly, our eyes and the skin around our eyes are the windows to our innermost thoughts and feelings.

# The underlying causes

AFTER YEARS OF SQUINTING IN THE SUN, LAUGHING, AND BLINKING, THE MUSCLES AROUND OUR EYES BECOME STRONGER. At the same time, the skin becomes thinner, making less collagen and ground substance. Periorbital eye skin is already thin, so time often reveals itself first around the eyes.

During the early stages of aging, periorbital changes can be hard to pinpoint. We subconsciously perceive the eye as older, yet it can be hard to say exactly why. Worse yet, we may perceive someone as angry, and not realize that it is because his or her eyebrows are always furrowed.

Dr. Richard Glogau developed a classification scheme to grade photoaging of the skin, and it can be applied to the periorbital skin to demonstrate the stepwise progression. You can compare your skin to the chart to see if your eyes and skin look older or younger than your true age.

## Glogau photoaging classification-wrinkle scale

| | |
|---|---|
| **Type I**<br>NO WRINKLES<br>PATIENT AGE 20S OR 30S | Mild pigmentary changes, no keratoses, minimal wrinkles. Minimal to no makeup needed. |
| **Type II**<br>WRINKLES IN MOTION<br>PATIENT AGE 30S OR 40S | Early lentigines (sun freckles or liver spots) visible, keratoses palpable but not visible, and parallel smile lines beginning to appear. Usually wears some foundation. |
| **Type III**<br>WRINKLES AT REST<br>PATIENT AGE 50 OR OLDER | Advanced photoaging, obvious pigment changes and telangiectasias, visible keratoses, wrinkles even when not moving facial muscles. Wears heavy foundation. |
| **Type IV**<br>ONLY WRINKLES<br>PATIENT AGE 60S TO 70S | Yellow-gray color of skin, prior skin cancers, and wrinkles throughout with no normal skin between. Can't wear makeup because it "cakes and cracks." |

# " Fran's story

I am a 71-year-old mother of three grown children and have nine grandchildren. I have been very active all my life, from publishing cookbooks to walking three miles five times a week and playing tennis whenever possible. Losing my wonderful husband five years ago in an accident has caused great stress to my being, showing up in my face most of all.

Needless to say, my appearance is important to me, as it is to most women. When you look your best, you feel your best.

I heard about the Fraxel re:pair® laser and felt it was a special opportunity for me to 'give it a shot.' I love the results! The wrinkles on my cheeks are much less deep and my brown spots mostly disappeared. My eyes appear brighter. The most amazing benefit is a glowing, radiant shine. I am so happy every time I wash my face! I've been told I look 50, not 70!

I was relaxed with a medicine and there was no pain for me. Afterward, you just take time off to relax and heal. The regimen after surgery is rigorous for 48 hours, but well worth it. No sun, period. Neutrogena® SPF 70 is my constant companion. You will be pleased. Be brave and go for it. It does make a difference."

AGE: 71
CONCERN: WRINKLES
TREATMENT: FRAXEL RE:PAIR LASER
NUMBER OF TREATMENTS: 1
DOWNTIME: 1 WEEK

BEFORE
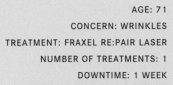
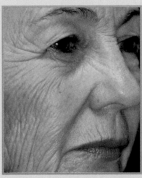

AFTER
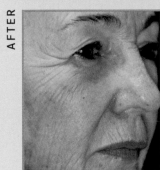

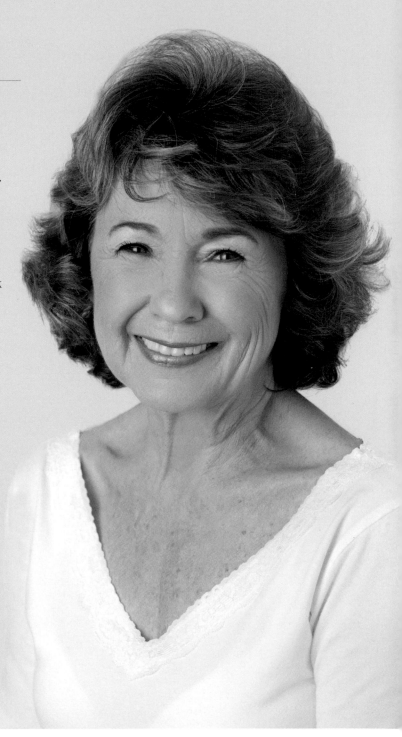

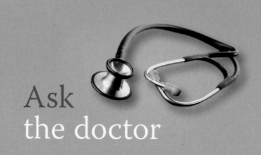

## WHAT CAUSES DARK CIRCLES AROUND MY EYES?

Dark circles can be caused by aging, hyperpigmentation from sun and genetics, or broken blood vessels. The skin under the eye becomes thinner as we age, allowing the blood vessels to become more visible and further contributing to darkness under the eyes. This is especially common for fair-skinned individuals. Also, fatigue, menopause, kidney, and thyroid disease can cause dark circles to appear.

Dark circles or blotches around the eyes can be treated with bleaching cream. However, upper and lower eyelid skin may be sensitive to these creams, making the creams best applied on the skin close to but not adjacent to the eye. Lasers remove pigment, broken blood vessels, and may improve fine lines.

# The underlying causes (continued)

ANOTHER WAY TO LOOK AT EYE AGING IS TO DETERMINE WHETHER THE PROBLEM IS THE THIN SKIN, THE UNDERLYING DERMIS, THE DEEPER MUSCLE, OR LESS COMMONLY THE FAT.

Thin skin is almost translucent and bluish, prompting the use of concealers. Or the skin can be a darker color, either from genetics, hormones, or sun. Hyperpigmentation all the way around the eyes creates "raccoon eyes." Hyperpigmentation just beneath the eyes creates "dark circles" or worsens hollows under the eyes. Those with darkness are perceived as being tired or sick. Dark triangles on the very tops of the cheeks and beneath the lower eyelids is called melasma. Commonly called the "mask of pregnancy," melasma may appear after pregnancy or with the use of oral contraceptives, but can also appear at any time and also in men. Underlying dermal volume loss from age results in sagging of the thin eyelid skin.

Furrowing your brows inward when upset strengthens the muscles just above and between the eyebrows. The corrugator and procerus muscles can become so thick they hood over the eye. This is subconsciously perceived as masculine, overbearing, and angry.

Use and hypertrophy of the muscle that encircles each eye eventually crinkles the overlying skin, creating crow's feet. At first these are cute laughter wrinkles, but later they can become deeply and permanently etched, collecting makeup and attention.

Normally there are small packets of fat all around the eye, secured into place by a thin septum. If the septum is thinned or breached, gravity can pull the fat down. This worsens and fills the "bags" above or below the eye. If the fat pad is contributing to lower or upper eyelid "bags," then surgery will be necessary for full correction. Surgery to remove fat and excess skin either above or below the eye is called blepharoplasty.

# Prevention and treatment options

EYELID SKIN IS THIN AND DELICATE. ANY CREAM, TREATMENT, OR PROCEDURE SHOULD BE ADJUSTED ACCORDINGLY. THE BEST THING TO DO IS WEAR SUNGLASSES AND SUNBLOCK. Clinique® makes a thick sunblock stick (like a large Chapstick®) that is less likely to sweat and drip down into the eyes. Sunblock will help prevent photoaging (thinning, pigmentation, and bumpiness). Eye creams containing antioxidants, moisturizers, and sunblock should be used to protect this tell-all area.

**SUNBLOCKS** can drip into the eyes and cause burning. Anything that doesn't normally irritate your skin can irritate the delicate and thin eyelid skin. If irritation is a problem, try sunblocks that contain only physical blockers like titanium dioxide or zinc oxide. Cost can range from $10 to $50, or even more, depending on the brand you choose. The more expensive brands may mix antioxidants and other age-combating ingredients into the same cream.

**PRESCRIPTION BLEACHING CREAMS AND RETINOIDS** should be used very sparingly and carefully around the eyes. Caution should be used to avoid any accidental application to the eye itself. Using too much will cause the delicate skin to be irritated, red, and itchy. In fact, it is recommended to apply these products only to the skin outside the periorbital rim, the bone that encircles the eye, from the eyebrow to below the lower lid.

Another treatment for dermal thinning and decreased collagen production is the injection of **DERMAL FILLERS**. The multitude of filler options is discussed in Chapter 3. Basically, a filler substance is injected into the dermis to replace any loss of tissue there. Restoring volume creates fullness and smoothes out overlying wrinkles. The use of fillers around the eye is not FDA-approved and should be done only by an experienced dermatologist, oculoplastic surgeon or facial plastic surgeon.

Dynamic wrinkles, or wrinkles that are a result of underlying muscle use, are treated with **BOTOX®** or **DYSPORT®**. Ideally, botulinum toxin should relax the muscles so that natural facial expression is still possible. Botulinum toxin is a protein that stops nerve endings from firing and stimulating muscle contraction.

**DOCTOR T!P**

After Botox® or Dysport® injections, consider contracting the muscles 15 times every 15 minutes for the next hour. This encourages the medicine to be taken up by the muscle.

It's the opposite with fillers. After filler injection, do not move or touch the treated area. The product is exactly where it belongs and should not be dislodged! Avoid dental procedures, facials, or other situations where someone might press down on your face for seven days.

# ❝ Lisa's story

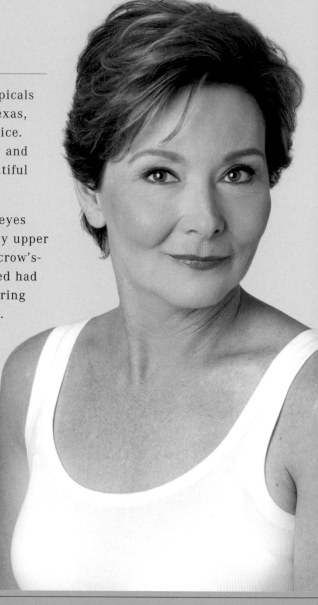

**AGE:** 46
**CONCERN:** WRINKLES, PHOTOAGING
**TREATMENT:** FRAXEL RE:PAIR LASER
**NUMBER OF TREATMENTS:** 1
**DOWNTIME:** 1 WEEK

**BEFORE**

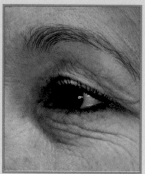

**AFTER**

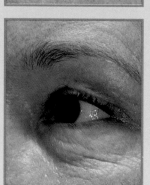

For several years I used Retin-A® and other prescription topicals and my skin looked fabulous. But after years of living in Texas, playing in the sun and smoking, my face was paying the price. I've been a nurse for over 20 years working in dermatology and surgery. My job revolves around helping patients look beautiful and have good skin day in and day out.

How can one sell beauty if one does not feel beautiful? My eyes especially bothered me. They used to be my best feature. My upper eyelids were sagging and sitting on my eyelashes, and my crow's-feet were deep and etching my face. The sun that I had loved had destroyed my looks. After debating the options and considering a facelift and going under the knife, I found Fraxel re:pair®. This was a better fit for me not only monetarily, but also because of the downtime associated with the procedure. I cannot afford to miss work for two weeks. And the cost of a facelift is not something attainable for a single mom.

The Fraxel re:pair® was the answer to my prayers. My face is gorgeous; I look great for my age and several years younger. I am now more confident at my job and in my personal life. My daughter was astounded and could not believe the results. I had not seen her in eight months; imagine her surprise when she walked through the door. That was a great feeling! After 10 years of being on my own, I am now engaged."

## PATIENT T!P

Bruising around the eye is very common. There are many tiny vessels around the eye, and the skin is thin. Avoid aspirin, ibuprofen, vitamin E, and alcohol for one week before and after any eye treatment. Ask your doctor before discontinuing any medications.

# Prevention and treatment options (continued)

**BOTOX® TREATMENT** involves multiple tiny injections around the wrinkled areas. Botox® comes as a powder in a vial, and is turned into a liquid for injection by mixing in sterile water. The amount of sterile water mixed in varies from physician to physician according to their preference. Cost should depend on the number of units used. Botox® is expensive even at wholesale cost. Price may range from $15 to $20 per unit.

Right after treatment with Botox®, you won't see any difference. You may see very tiny injection sites, which will heal in a few hours. Most patients can go back to work immediately. It may take up to two weeks to see the full effect. If at two weeks you feel the treatment is uneven or you desire more, your provider can do touch-ups.

After the injection of Botox®, the muscles treated will be relaxed for about four months. Depending on how strong your muscles are and how frequently you use them, the treatment will last a little shorter or longer. The number of units (not the actual volume amount) of Botox® used also determines duration.

**DYSPORT®**, another brand of botulinum toxin type A, was recently approved by the FDA. This product works in the same manner as Botox®, and cost is typically determined by the number of units used.

Pigment-removing **LASERS** include the Q-switched Nd:YAG, Q-switched ruby and Q-switched alexandrite. Pigment lasers work by breaking up pigment molecules so they are able to be cleared by your immune system.

**INTENSE PULSED LIGHT SOURCES** can also be used to treat pigmentation, wrinkles, and telangiectasias around the eyes from sun damage.

# Prevention and treatment options (continued)

Fractionated lasers improve both pigment and wrinkles. The new fractionated carbon dioxide lasers result in better and quicker improvements, with less downtime as compared to ablative lasers. Ablative lasers like carbon dioxide and Er:YAG improve skin pigment and texture dramatically, but expect a week of downtime and risks for infection, scarring, and hypopigmentation. Lasers for wrinkles work by heating collagen and stimulating collagen formation.

**NON-ABLATIVE LASER TREATMENT** will result in minimal redness and swelling of the treated area. During the treatment, the eyes will be protected with appropriate eye protection. If the eyelid itself is being treated, a protective shield is inserted like a contact lens onto the eye. Non-ablative fractional laser treatments may cause marked redness and swelling lasting one to two days. Multiple monthly sessions will be needed. Cost for treating just the eyes will be less than treating the whole face, perhaps about $500 per session. After a series of treatments, the effect should be permanent, with the caveat that aging continues and treatment does not prevent that process. Pigment, however, can quickly return, especially if there is a sun or hormonal cause. It is imperative to wear sunblock after treatment to maintain the benefits.

**ABLATIVE LASER TREATMENT** of the eyelids will yield raw, moist, and pink skin. Keep the area slathered in Vaseline® or petrolatum ointment, as directed by your provider. Again, the skin here is thin, so it heals faster than the rest of your face, perhaps in one week. Plan to take off work for a week; you will be raw and swollen. Most patients experience at least a 50 percent improvement in pigment and wrinkles after only one treatment. If you have a history

**PATIENT T!P**

Cooling reduces swelling. Cold compresses, refrigerated gels and cooling masks relieve morning puffiness.

of herpes simplex virus (fever blisters or cold sores), you should be prescribed antiviral medications to prevent infection of the treated skin. Given the higher risk and need for perioperative medications and monitoring, one ablative treatment will cost more than a non-ablative laser treatment. Prices for laser treatment varies, especially if used in combination with blepharoplasty, but may range from $2,000 to $5,000. Results should be permanent. Very few patients will require another treatment several years later.

Advanced sagging from fat pad dislocation can be masked by the use of fillers or improving the texture of overlying skin. However, full improvement of the sagging or bags will require a small incision and removal of the fat. The incision can be made with a scalpel or laser. This type of procedure can be performed on the upper eyelids and/or the lower eyelids and is called an upper or lower blepharoplasty. A simpler type of blepharoplasty removes excess skin and not fat. For this procedure, seek an experienced physician, such as a plastic surgeon, oculoplastic surgeon, or dermatologic surgeon.

For **BLEPHAROPLASTY**, the incision is usually hidden in the crease above the eye, on the eyelash rim below the eye, or just inside the lower eyelid. The incision above the eye is usually closed with tiny stitches that need to be removed in five to seven days. Other incisions may be closed with stitches that need to be removed or stitches that dissolve. Swelling and a little redness is expected for a few days. Bruising is common and may last for two weeks. The effects of a blepharoplasty are, for the most part, permanent.

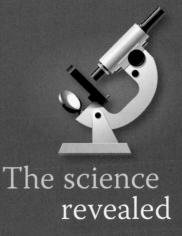

## The science revealed

HYALURONIC ACID DERMAL FILLERS CAN BE USED TO RESTORE VOLUME IN THE TEAR TROUGHS.

If product is placed too superficially it can result in a bluish discoloration of the skin known as the "Tyndall effect." Hyaluronidase is an enzyme that degrades hyaluronic acid and can be used by your physician to correct this unwanted side effect.

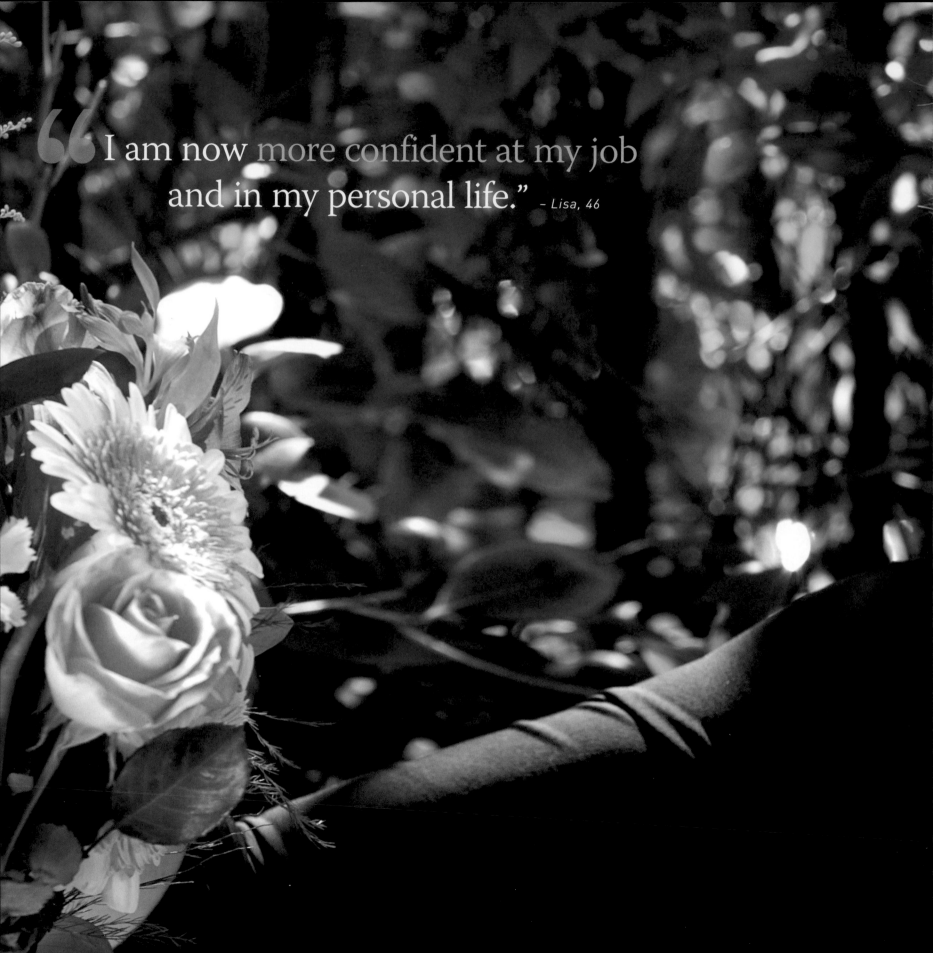

"I am now more confident at my job and in my personal life." – Lisa, 46

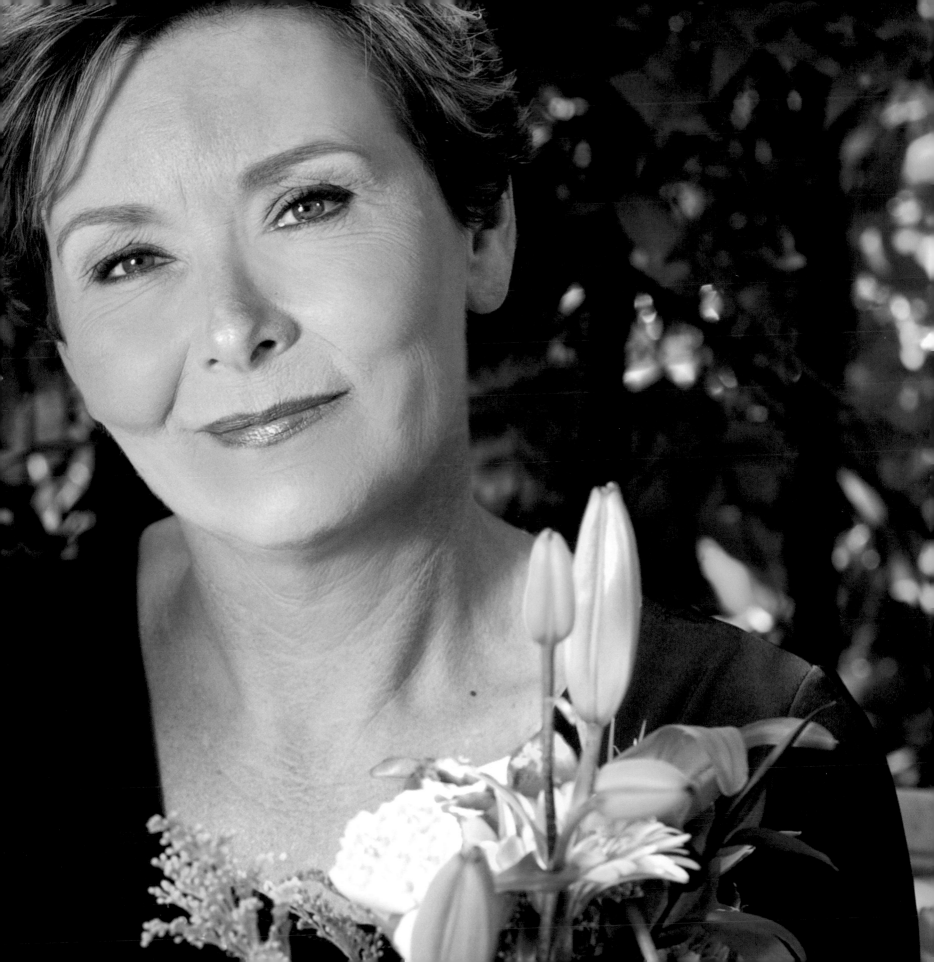

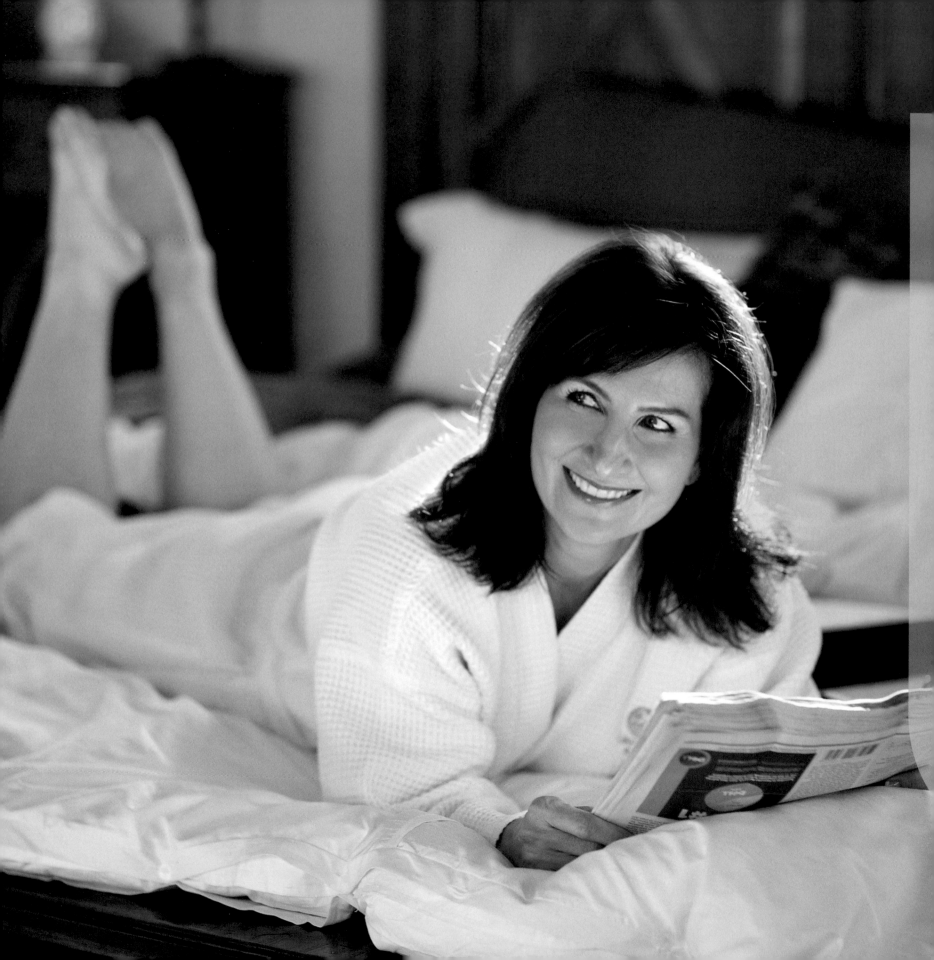

# CHAPTER 7

# LEG VEINS

> ❝I've always been self-conscious about the spider veins ON MY LEGS.'"
>
> – *Kathryn, 46*

Do you dread warm weather because you don't want the world to see your leg veins? Does it seem your days of shorts and mini-skirts are over? Visible veins on the legs are a common concern, affecting 80 percent of women in the United States. Spider veins can become more prominent as we age and with jobs requiring prolonged standing. Pregnancy causes increased pressure in the venous system, which can lead to varicose veins. Several techniques are available to reduce the appearance of veins.

# Why it occurs

THE LEGS HAVE BOTH SUPERFICIAL AND DEEP VEINS. The superficial venous system lies in the fat below the skin. These veins connect to perforating veins that extend deeper into the leg and connect to the deep venous system in the muscle below.

One-way valves direct the flow of venous blood upward and inward to the deeper veins, up the legs, and eventually to the heart. Aging, genetics, hormones, pregnancy, upright posture, and trauma can contribute to failure of the venous valves, resulting in backflow. The blood then leaks from the deep veins backward to the lower-pressure superficial veins. The superficial veins bulge with all the pooled blood, becoming visible through the skin.

Dilations of the most superficial and tiny veins are called telangiectasias. These are usually bright red, fine lines. Slightly larger are red or blue venulectasias. Telangiectasis and venulectasias are commonly referred to as spider veins. These connect to larger and deeper reticular veins that appear blue because of their depth. Varicose veins are even deeper veins that drain into the superficial venous system.

Aside from seeing red or blue lines, or deep blue cords, you may also experience pain, burning, muscle fatigue, cramping, and restless legs. Symptoms may worsen with heat, menses, pregnancy, oral contraceptive use, or hormone replacement therapy. Symptoms may be severe, even if it appears the veins are small. Over time, backward flow of blood results in chronic venous insufficiency, seen as swelling, hyperpigmented spots, rashes, and ulcers.

## PATIENT T!P

When the long-pulsed Nd:YAG laser or sclerotherapy is used to treat vessels greater than 2 mm in diameter, local clot formation may occur. Compression garments should be used following laser treatments of leg veins, as with sclerotherapy.

# Kathryn's story

After three rounds of sclerotherapy, I still had very small spider veins, which were not large enough to be corrected by additional sclerotherapy, on both legs.

My dermatologist recommended the Altus laser, and after two treatments I had excellent results. The veins on the right leg all but disappeared, but some smaller veins on my left leg still remained.

AGE: 46
CONCERN: LEG VEINS
TREATMENT: SCLEROTHERAPY, ALTUS AND VBEAM LASERS
NUMBER OF TREATMENTS: 4
DOWNTIME: COMPRESSION STOCKINGS FOR 2-3 WEEKS

Since I was concerned about the potential risk of hyperpigmentation (brown spots) but still wanted to rid my legs of the few remaining small spider veins, my dermatologist treated me with the Vbeam laser at modified settings. We always did a small test area, and there was never a sign of hyperpigmentation. After my procedures, the sites always healed quickly.

Overall, I have been extremely pleased with my results. I highly recommend a combination of sclerotherapy and laser therapies to others with spider veins. The treatments are relatively painless, and they provide great results! Having legs free of spider veins makes a big difference in what I can wear and how I feel."

BEFORE

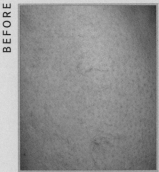

AFTER

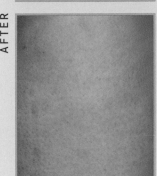

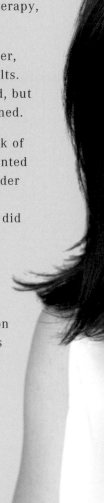

# Treatment options and how they work

THE DEVELOPMENT OF VARICOSE VEINS CAN BE PREVENTED OR SLOWED BY WEARING COMPRESSION STOCKINGS. Medical grade compression stockings list the amount of pressure (tightness) on the label. These typically come in low, medium, and high strengths. Healthy individuals wishing to prevent disease or those having only slight disease should wear the 15-20 mmHg strength. You can choose knee-high, thigh-high, or full-length stocking styles. Most women develop varicose veins not only along the ankle, but behind the knee and on the lower thigh, so thigh-high or full length are the best. Stockings should be worn for the entire day, or at least during times when you'll be standing for prolonged periods. By applying external pressure on the leg, the stockings massage the leg to encourage normal blood flow.

Spider veins and reticular veins are best treated with **sclerotherapy**. This involves the injection of a sclerosing solution directly in the vein. The sclerosing solution causes the vein to squeeze closed. Wearing compression stockings for two weeks after treatment helps the vein stay closed.

For those who do not like needles, or have not had a good response to sclerotherapy, lasers can be used to treat spider veins. The combination of sclerotherapy and laser therapy is quite effective. The **pulsed-dye laser** is used for the most superficial and tiny veins, whereas the **long-pulsed Nd:YAG** or **long-pulsed alexandrite** is used for slightly deeper veins. Laser treatment will not be effective for very deep or bulging veins.

The laser works by heating the blood, which in turn heats the surrounding vessel. The vessel contracts and heals in the closed position. Alternatively coagulated blood may form a clot and permanently block the vein. The inflammation process that follows eventually destroys the vessel. Compression stockings are worn for two weeks after treatment to encourage the veins to stay closed.

During your first consultation visit, you may have a Doppler ultrasound examination performed. This involves cool jelly being placed on the leg, and a small imaging wand being pressed against the leg. The amount of bumpy unpleasing veins seen on the surface of the skin does not mean there will or will not be deeper vein incompetence. However, an ultrasound is often recommended to search for deeper venous disease, especially if the patient is symptomatic.

If backflow is also occurring in larger varicose veins and superficial venous system veins, then these larger vessels should be treated first. Treating the tiny spider veins without treating underlying deeper vein backflow can be done, but results are unlikely to last for more than a couple of years.

Deeper veins are treated with **phlebectomy** or **endovenous therapy**. Phlebectomy, or vein stripping, involves small incisions to pull the diseased vein out. Endovenous therapy involves the insertion of a small laser or radioablative device through the skin and into the vein. From inside the vein, heat is applied to the surrounding vessel wall and induces collagen contraction. After the vein wall contracts, the device is withdrawn a few inches. This is repeated several times until the entire diseased vein is heated and contracted.

Phlebectomy and endovenous therapy are both outpatient procedures. Very tight wraps are worn for one week. Then compression stockings are worn for another three weeks. A repeat ultrasound is performed three weeks after treatment to see if the veins have remained closed and also to make sure that clots have not formed. After deep veins are treated in this manner, smaller veins can be treated with injections or laser.

# Sclerotherapy
# questions and answers

**Q: WHEN CAN I START WALKING?**
Immediately! In fact it's good to walk right away. Avoid aerobic exercise, weight training, and any other activity that may increase your breathing and pulse rate for one week.

**Q: WHEN CAN I RETURN TO WORK?**
You can work the next day, depending on your job.

**Q: HOW LONG DO I NEED TO WEAR THE COMPRESSION STOCKINGS?**
The stockings are there to make sure the veins stay closed. Wear them during the day for at least two weeks after the procedure.

**Q: WHAT OTHER RESTRICTIONS ARE THERE?**
Do not drink alcohol for two days after the procedure. Do not go into a hot tub for one week after the procedure.

**Q: IF I HAVE PAIN, WHAT CAN I TAKE?**
The pain is much less than getting your blood drawn. You should not need medication after treatment. You may take Tylenol® as directed on the box. If this does not completely resolve your discomfort, contact your physician. Do not take aspirin or ibuprofen for five days after your procedure, unless approved by your physician.

**Q: WHAT ARE THE POSSIBLE SIDE EFFECTS?**
Side effects include bruising, swelling, brownish staining, darkening of the treated veins, and small clotted vessels under the surface of the skin.

**Q: WHEN SHOULD I SEEK MEDICAL ATTENTION?**
If you have a fever, increasing redness or pain, drainage of pus, or pain not relieved by Tylenol, you should seek medical attention. Also, you should call your doctor if you experience continuous bleeding from injection sites, injection sites that turn black or ulcerate, or if blisters develop.

# What to expect (risks, cost, duration)

JOBST® BRAND MEDICAL-GRADE STOCKINGS COST ABOUT $60 PER PAIR. WITH DAILY USE, A PAIR CAN BE EXPECTED TO LAST SIX MONTHS. At first, it is recommended to try a lower compression grade, like 8–15 mmHg for a month, until you get used to the "tightness" of the stockings.

Lower and medium strength compression stockings are generally not associated with any side effects. However, patients with severe vein disease, peripheral vascular disease, poor circulation, or other blood problems should consult their physician before buying a pair. In these patients, tight constriction can prevent blood flow and exacerbate disease.

Sclerotherapy involves multiple small injections using an agent that irritates the veins. The needle used is tiny, and is inserted just below the skin, so the pain is minimal. In most studies, patients actually prefer the pain associated with the needle prick over the pain from a quick laser blast.

Depending on the solution used, you may or may not feel heat and cramping as it is injected. The number of veins that can be treated in a given session is limited by the amount of sclerosant that can be injected at any one time. If there are multiple veins, then multiple sessions may be needed. Expect about a 50 percent improvement after each treatment. Treatments are continued until the desired clinical end point is achieved.

Laser treatment involves aiming the laser beam directly at the vessel. The laser is fired or pulsed along the vessel. You'll feel a quick burst, like a rubber band snapping, each time the laser is fired. There may be bruising along the treated sites, and this will fade over two weeks. Patients with dark skin may have hyperpigmentation in the treated areas for a few months.

With local anesthesia and a calming oral medication, phlebectomy and endovenous ablation are usually well-tolerated.

## PATIENT T!P

If it is not prescribed by a physician, then do not take aspirin, ibuprofen, or other nonsteroidal anti-inflammatory drugs for five days after your treatment, as this may increase bruising.

# Approximate costs

| | |
|---|---|
| Laser therapy | $500 per treatment session, multiple sessions needed |
| Sclerotherapy | $500 per treatment session, multiple sessions needed |
| Duplex guided sclerotherapy for larger veins | $1000 per treatment |
| Outpatient phlebectomy | $1500–$3000 per session (one thigh or lower leg per session) |
| Outpatient endovenous ablation | $3000–$5000 per leg |

# Sclerotherapy or laser treatment checklist

✓ EAT A LIGHT MEAL OR SNACK PRIOR TO YOUR APPOINTMENT.

✓ BRING LOOSE FITTING SHORTS TO WEAR DURING THE TREATMENT.

✓ BRING TWO PAIRS OF COMPRESSION STOCKINGS AND WEAR STOCKINGS 24 HOURS PER DAY FOR THREE TO FIVE DAYS.

✓ USE SHOWER BAGS OVER THE STOCKINGS DURING SHOWERS.

✓ CONTINUE TO WEAR STOCKINGS DURING THE DAYTIME FOR AN ADDITIONAL THREE WEEKS.

✓ AVOID ALCOHOLIC BEVERAGES FOR TWO DAYS AFTER YOUR TREATMENT AS THIS MAY IMPAIR HEALING.

BEFORE

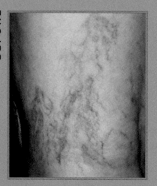

AFTER

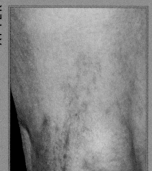

# Guide to light and laser treatments

| Treatment type | Brand options | Best for | Treatments |
| --- | --- | --- | --- |
| Pulsed-dye Laser | Candela® (Vbeam®, Vbeam® Perfecta) | Tiny red spider veins in fair skin | Feels like a rubber band snapping against your skin |
| Intense Pulsed Light | Cutera® (CoolGlide® Xeo), Palomar (StarLux®) | Superficial spider veins | May require 1 hour of topical anesthesia before treatment |
| Long-pulsed Alexandrite Laser | Candela® (GentleLase®), Cynosure® (Apogee™) | Medium-sized vessels | Cooling techniques are used to reduce discomfort and enable higher energy to be utilized |
| Long-pulsed Nd:YAG Laser | Cutera® (CoolGlide® Vantage), Laserscope (Lyra™), Candela® (GentleYAG®), Sciton (Profile™), CoolTouch® (Varia™) | Most leg veins up to 3 mm in diameter | Active skin cooling will be used during treatment |

| Recovery | Follow up visit | Tips |
|---|---|---|
| Bruising can last from 2 days to 2 weeks. Transient hyperpigmentation. | 4–6 weeks, requires several treatments | *Avoid aspirin, vitamin E, caffeine, and alcohol 5 days before and after the procedure to reduce bruising. Apply ice to halt bruise formation. |
| Redness or swelling may develop. Recommend no exercise for 24 hours. | 2–4 weeks, requires several treatments | Sun-tanned skin can not be treated with this device. Avoid sun exposure prior to and after treatment. |
| Bruising, redness, crusting, and hyperpigmentation may occur and typically resolves over 3 months | 4 weeks, requires several treatments | Telangiectatic matting may be a side effect of this treatment |
| Mild to moderate redness and swelling resolve within 48–72 hrs | 6–8 weeks, requires several treatments | Application of a topical anesthetic cream prior to treatment may be beneficial |

*Please consult your physician before discontinuing any medication.

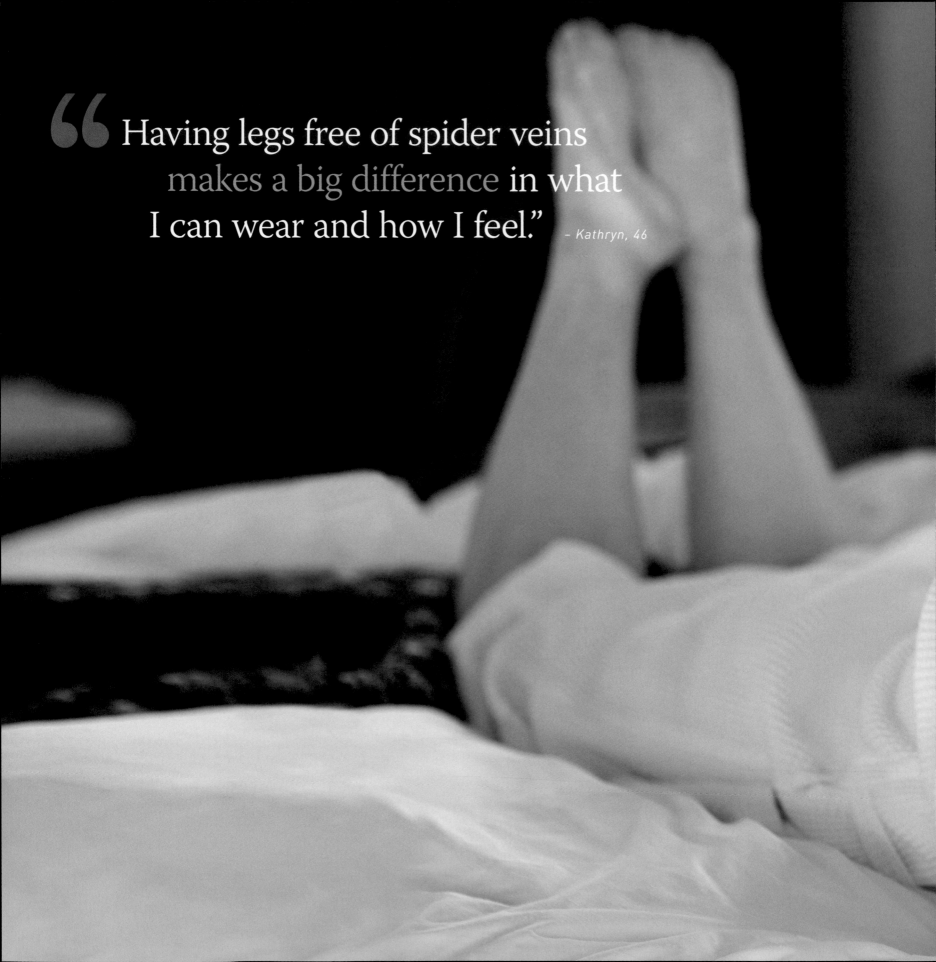

> " Having legs free of spider veins
> makes a big difference in what
> I can wear and how I feel." – *Kathryn, 46*

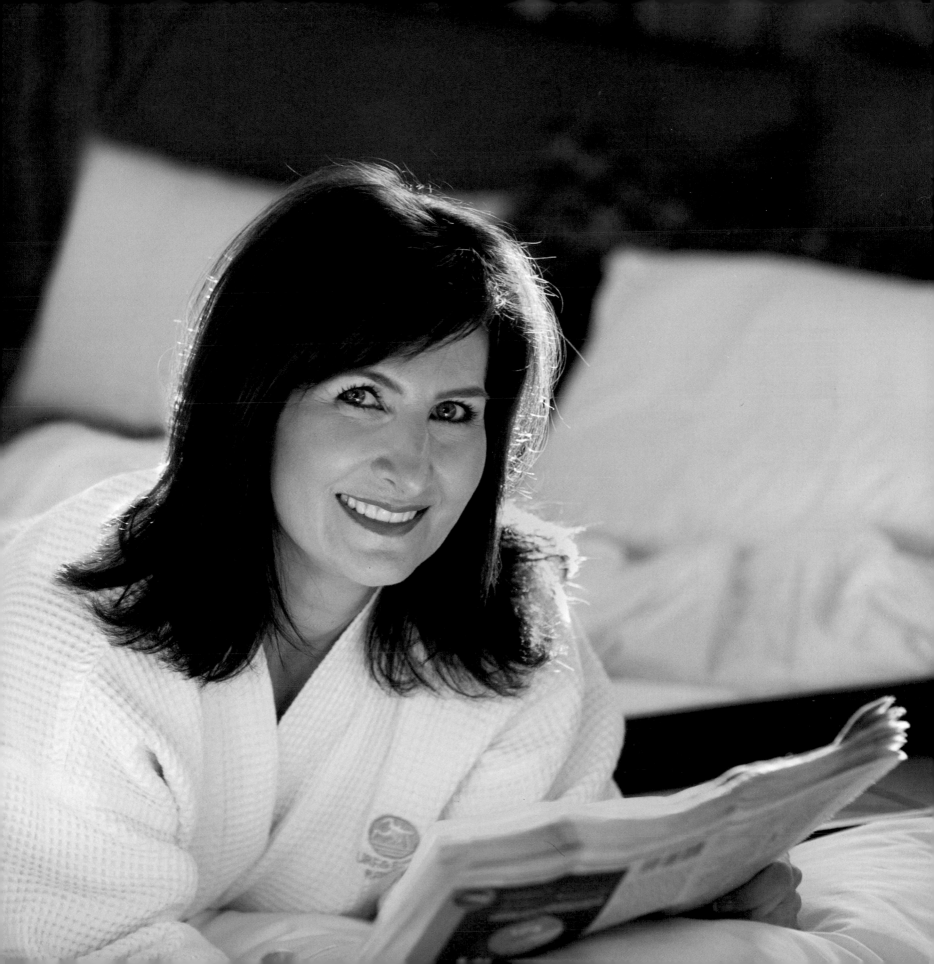

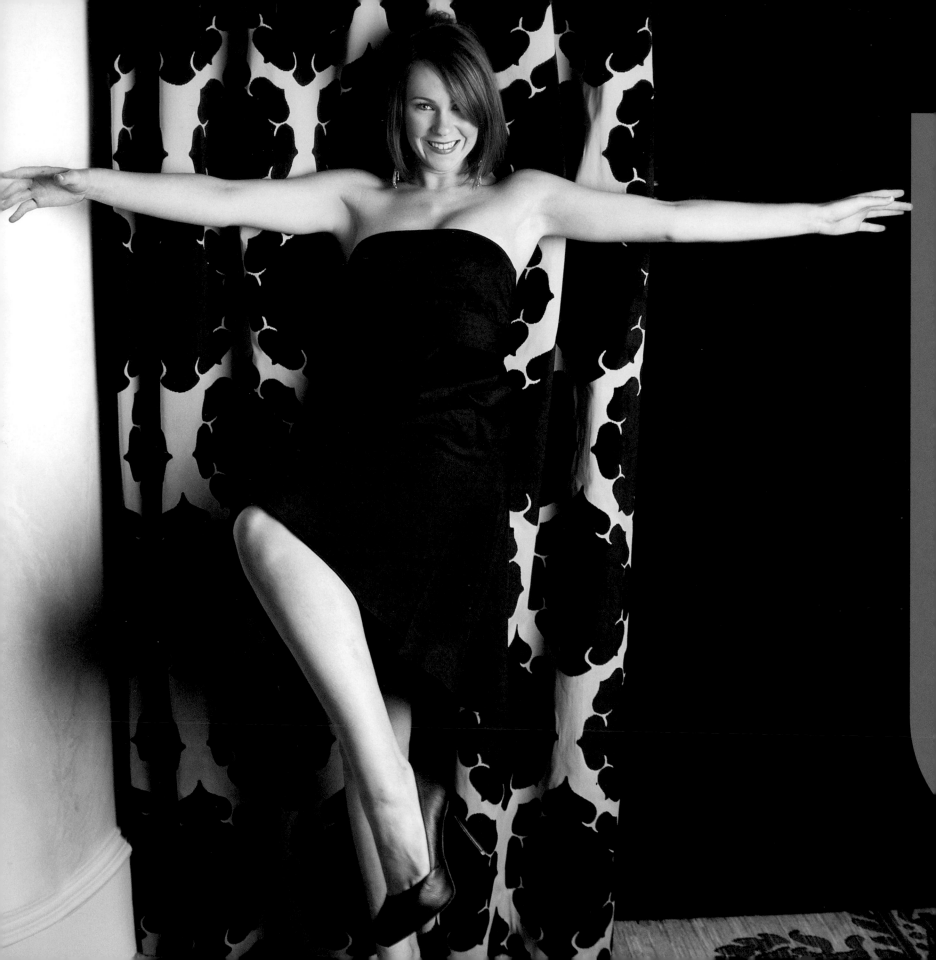

# CHAPTER 8

# SKIN CANCER

> " Hearing the word 'cancer' is always scary,
>
> **AND IT'S ESPECIALLY SCARY WHEN THEY SAY YOU ARE THE ONE WHO HAS IT!"**
>
> *– Taylor, 18*

Can a sunny disposition get you in trouble? Sun can significantly accelerate the rate at which you appear to age. Brown spots, wrinkles, leathery skin, and hyperpigmentation are all caused by the sun. Still can't give up that sun-kissed look? Consider this: skin cancers occur more frequently than all other types of cancer combined. The most common kind of skin cancer, basal cell cancer, affects 1 million Americans each year. The most serious kind of skin cancer, melanoma, is on the rise. There are 80,000 new cases of melanoma every year.

Skin cancers are a progression, resulting from an accumulation of sun damage and mutations. So, you can still prevent the sun damage you see today from becoming skin cancer tomorrow.

# Taylor's story

My whole life I have always played outside at the beach and swam at the pool on the swim team. I would never wear sunscreen because I thought I looked better with a tan. I even used tanning beds. Both of my parents also used tanning beds to 'keep color.' The harmful effects of the sun were never discussed in my family, mostly because we were uneducated about it. Until recently, skin cancer had never been taken seriously in my family.

At the age of 18, I was diagnosed with malignant melanoma—the deadliest and most serious form of skin cancer. I originally went to my dermatologist for acne and then casually mentioned a dark but normal-shaped freckle on my left leg. The dermatologist ended up removing the freckle and sent it in for microscopic examination. About a week later I received news that the freckle was malignant melanoma, and I needed to have surgery as soon as possible. The surgery took about an hour. The surgeon made an incision of about 3 inches long and 1 inch wide. After the surgery I was left with an indentation in my leg and a 3-inch-long red scar. My doctor recommended Fraxel® treatments to reduce the scar. After three treatments, the redness of my scar was completely gone and the texture greatly improved.

I am now an avid spokesperson for skin cancer awareness. I wear sunscreen every day and have not touched a tanning bed since my diagnosis. I am now very aware of the harmful and deadly effects of the sun and use precautionary measures. My experience has been an eye-opener for my family and friends. I still continue to enjoy the same hobbies and interests but with sun protection."

AGE: 18
CONCERN: MELANOMA IN-SITU
TREATMENT: EXCISION
DOWNTIME: 2 WEEKS

BEFORE

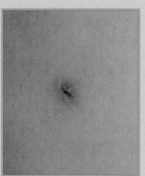

AFTER

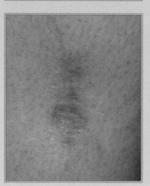

# Prevention

SKIN CANCER IS HIGHLY PREVENTABLE IF YOU SIMPLY AVOID THE SUN DURING PEAK HOURS AND APPLY SUNBLOCK. Remember the problem is UV light, not visible light. So even on a cloudy and dark day, UV light from the sun penetrates through clouds. Use these sun-sensible tips:

▸ Avoid sun during peak hours (10 a.m. to 4 p.m.) when the sun is strongest and does the most damage. Apply sunblock every four hours.

▸ Avoid tanning booths. Tanning booths concentrate the light, so you will burn faster. You'll get mainly UVA, which causes photoaging and has been linked to melanoma. The World Health Organization has moved UV tanning beds to its highest cancer risk category—"carcinogenic to humans." The risk of skin cancer increases by 75 percent when people begin using tanning beds prior to age 30.

▸ Wear sun protective clothing with a UPF rating. Note that a plain white shirt only has UPF 3, so you might as well be naked! You can buy clothes with a UPF rating online or at sporting goods stores. Adding a colorless dye like Rit® Sun Guard to the laundry can coat the fibers of your existing wardrobe, giving regular clothes SPF 30.

▸ The newest sunscreens promise SPF 50 or above, but you may be surprised to learn the American Academy of Dermatology recommends SPF 30. SPF measures how much longer you can stay out in the sun, before getting a little pink. If SPF 30 sunscreen is applied liberally, you should be able to stay out in the sun 30 times longer before seeing any signs of pink. The problem lies in the amount of product applied. Most people don't use nearly enough often enough, so you're getting far less protection than the bottle says. It takes one tablespoon for the face, and a full shot glass for the body and must be reapplied every four hours, more often if swimming or perspiring. Even if you feel the greasy sunblock is still on your skin, the particles that absorb light have been used and more needs to be applied. Use a sunscreen that blocks both UVA and UVB light. SPF tells you the amount of UVB blockage. There is no rating system for UVA blockage at this time, so look for ingredients that block UVA light (ecamsule or mexoryl, avobenzone (Parsol 1789) and oxybenzone (Helioplex), titanium dioxide, zinc oxide, iron oxide).

▸ It's a good idea to apply 30 minutes before sun exposure. UV protection increases with higher SPF numbers, but after a point, it really doesn't help that much...the benefits level off. That's why your doctor will most likely recommend SPF 30. The bottom line is that SPF ratings are based on applying lots of cream repeatedly throughout the day. Ask your dermatologist what SPF is right for you.

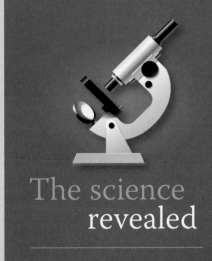

## The science revealed

THE SUN AND VITAMIN D HAVE STIRRED UP QUITE A CONTROVERSY: It is true that vitamin D is important and needed for bone formation and the immune system. It may even have a role in fighting cancer and diabetes.

However, how much vitamin D your body really needs is not yet known. It is estimated that most healthy people need an amount equal to what is contained in one glass of milk or other serving of dairy. If you don't eat dairy, five to 10 minutes of sun is enough to make adequate vitamin D. Taking Vitamin D supplements may be appropriate, depending upon your overall health. Purposeful tanning and prolonged sun exposure will increase your risk for skin cancer.

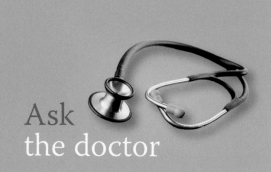

## Ask the doctor

# What are the different types of skin cancer?

LET'S TAKE A CLOSER LOOK AT SKIN CANCER. THERE ARE THREE MAIN TYPES OF SKIN CANCER: BASAL CELL CANCER, SQUAMOUS CELL CANCER, AND MELANOMA. THE TYPE OF CANCER IS DETERMINED BY THE SPECIFIC CELL TYPE INVOLVED. For instance, when the cells that line the colon grow uncontrollably, you get colon cancer. When the cells that make up the epidermis (keratinocytes) proliferate, you get squamous cell cancer. When the cells that make up the lower part of the epidermis proliferate, you develop basal cell cancer. When the pigment cells called melanocytes proliferate, you get melanoma.

Melanoma is the most serious of the three types of skin cancer. The most important thing to know about melanoma is the depth. A thin melanoma that has not grown downward into the skin can be cut out. Once excised, there is essentially a 99 percent cure rate and normal life expectancy. If the melanoma is diagnosed after it has already grown deeply, the prognosis is less optimistic.

"Lentigo maligna" is a melanoma in situ on sun-damaged skin. This means the melanoma cells are constricted to the top layer of skin, the epidermis. This is not the same as a "lentigo maligna melanoma," which is a true melanoma. It is more likely that the melanoma will spread to other sites.

ACTINIC KERATOSIS

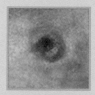

BASAL CELL CARCINOMA

SQUAMOUS CELL CARCINOMA

MELANOMA

**MORE ABOUT PRE-CANCERS AND SQUAMOUS CELL CANCER**. Actinic keratoses are very common pre-cancers, affecting 11 percent to 26 percent of persons over age 40. They look like small red bumps with a scale. They can often be felt more easily than seen. They can be a discrete bump, or ill-defined red, scaly splotches scattered over the skin's surface.

Since approximately one in every 12 actinic keratoses will become squamous cell cancer, actinic keratoses should be treated. In some patients, aggressive monitoring and treatment is necessary. Patients who smoke or take immune-suppressing medications have a higher chance of progression to cancer. And the progression itself can be faster.

Squamous cell cancer is usually superficial—just within the top layers of the skin. Once it is cut out, it is considered "cured." However, about 5 percent of squamous cell cancers spread to other parts of the body, and can be fatal. Cancers on the lips and around the nose, eyes, or ears tend to be more aggressive.

Sun exposure, fair skin, smoking, lymphoma, longstanding wounds and immunosuppression from drugs or disease are all risk factors for developing a squamous cell cancer. Squamous cell cancer is not hereditary in and of itself, but if you inherited fair skin your risk is increased.

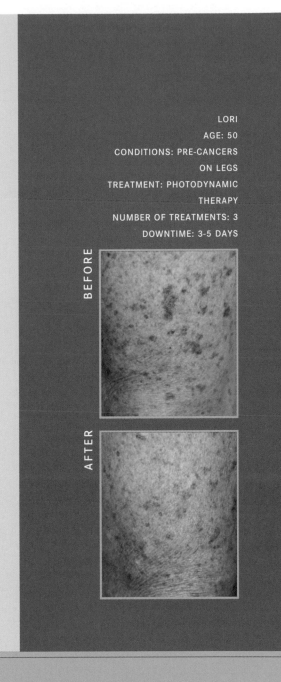

LORI
AGE: 50
CONDITIONS: PRE-CANCERS
ON LEGS
TREATMENT: PHOTODYNAMIC
THERAPY
NUMBER OF TREATMENTS: 3
DOWNTIME: 3-5 DAYS

BEFORE

AFTER

**PATIENT T!P**

If you have significant past sun exposure or a family history of skin cancer, it's a good idea to have an annual skin examination by a dermatologist.

## Specific signs of melanoma

**SIGNS THAT A MOLE MAY BE MELANOMA (ABCDEs):**

**ASYMMETRY**

**BORDER IRREGULAR OR SCALLOPED** (should be a smooth circle) OR **BORDER THAT CHANGES** (shape of mole should remain the same)

**COLOR** (more than two colors, i.e. red, blue, and brown)

**DIAMETER GREATER THAN** a pencil eraser or darker

**EVOLVING** (any change in size, height, color or symptoms like itching, burning, pain, or bleeding)

**UGLY DUCKLING** (mole that looks different from all your other moles)

**RISK FACTORS FOR MELANOMA:**

**FAIR SKIN**

**RED HAIR**

**SUN EXPOSURE**

**SUNBURNS**

**MORE THAN 50 MOLES**

**FAMILY HISTORY OF MELANOMA**

*Patients with risk factors should undergo regular skin screening exams by a dermatologist.*

## What are the different types of skin cancer? (continued)

**MORE ABOUT BASAL CELL CANCER**. The most common type of skin cancer is basal cell cancer. Basal cell cancer has the best prognosis of the three main types of skin cancer because it usually stays in the skin. Less than 1 percent of basal cell cancers ever metastasize or (spread to other parts of the body). Although they don't have the tendency to metastasize, they still require treatment because they can grow wider and deeper, destroying surrounding structures.

Risk factors for developing basal cell cancer are sun exposure, fair skin, smoking, immunosuppression, and arsenic exposure.

**MORE ABOUT MELANOMA**. How do I know if a mole is really melanoma? Most patients believe that moles are the primary focus of melanoma, but only one third of melanomas arise in moles. You can think of moles and melanoma as being part of a spectrum. On the benign side you have regular moles. On the malignant side you have melanoma cancer. In the middle you have moles with atypical features. These uncommon features can be graded as mild, moderate, or severe. It's important to recognize that a strange mole, called a dysplastic nevus, will most likely stay just a strange, but benign mole. Though benign, severe dysplastic nevi will often need to be excised.

Again, the most important prognostic factor is depth. A melanoma that has grown more than 1 mm thick (about as thick as a Sharpie marker line) has a higher likelihood of spreading to other parts of the body, usually the nearest lymph node. Early detection is critical. If the melanoma is thick or has spread to another part of the body, the result is a less favorable prognosis.

# Lynell's story

For years, I was not as conscientious about skin care as I should have been. Among other mistakes, I exposed my skin to too much sun. When I was growing up, we used iodine in baby oil to get the darkest possible tan!

In my 30s, I had a basal cell cancer removed. I knew I needed to start taking care of my skin, and for a while I stayed out of the sun. But my memories of cancer faded, and I started going to a tanning bed.

Then when I was 48, I found an unusual freckle on my chest. I asked my regular physician about it, and he told me not to worry about it. But when I visited my dermatologist to see if laser treatment would help my sun-damaged skin, he biopsied the spot. Three days later, I found out it was melanoma.

After that, everything happened so fast. I had Mohs micrographic surgery to remove the spot and the surrounding skin. The entire perimeter was checked for cancer cells while I waited in the office. By the end of the day, the area was free of cancer cells. Finding the cancer early, before it had spread, probably saved my life.

Now, I wear sunscreen every day and watch my skin for any changes. My years of too much sun will always increase my chances for skin cancer, but with yearly examinations I can lessen the chances of it being life threatening. And with the new laser technology available, I can keep my skin looking fresh and healthy for a long time."

AGE: 50
CONCERN: MELANOMA
TREATMENT: WIDE
LOCAL EXCISION
DOWNTIME: LESS THAN 1 WEEK

**BEFORE**

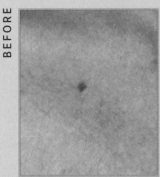

**AFTER**

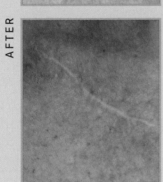

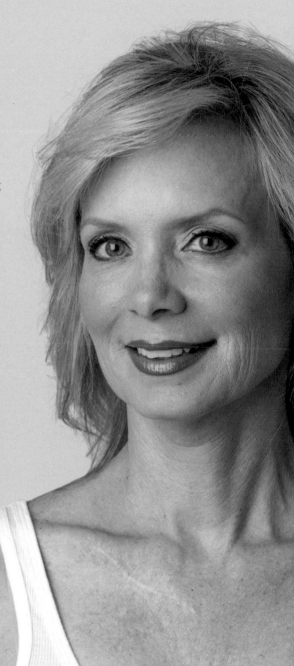

# Treatments options for actinic keratoses and skin cancer

| Treatment | How it's done |
|---|---|
| Cryotherapy | Very cold liquid nitrogen is sprayed onto the lesion |
| Efudex® cream | Cream is applied to area with actinic keratoses twice a day, for 2 weeks |
| Carac® cream | Cream is applied to area with actinic keratoses once a day, for 4 weeks |
| Aldara® cream | Cream is applied to precancerous area 3 times a week for 6–8 weeks. Other dosing schedules are popular. |
| Solaraze™ cream | Cream is applied twice a day for 60–90 days |
| Photodynamic therapy | Photosensitizer applied to the actinic keratoses for 1–3 hours followed by illumination with a high-intensity light or laser |
| Curretage & Electrodessication | Physician scrapes the cancer away, then burns the base. The procedure is repeated 1–2 times. Burnt area is allowed to heal on its own. |
| Excision | Tumor and some surrounding normal skin are removed. For a simple lesion, extra triangles of skin need to be removed in order to sew the skin closed with a straight line. |
| Wide local excision | Tumor and usually 1 cm or more of normal surrounding skin is excised |
| Mohs surgery | Only the tumor is removed. All edges are mapped and examined with a microscope. If any tumor is seen at the border, then more skin is removed incrementally. |
| Radiation | Radiation beams focus on the tumor. May increase risk for skin cancer and other cancers long term. Typically used for patients who are not surgical candidates, or as part of the treatment plan for squamous cell carcinoma or melanoma. |
| Interferon injections | Injections of clear fluid placed around the entire tumor. Efficacy is lower than excision, and advised only where patient declares scarring cannot be tolerated. Patient must be willing to accept cancer may grow back. |
| Interferon intramuscular injections | Used as an additional treatment for some melanoma patients |

## Time to heal

May blister 3 days later, heals in 1–2 weeks

During the second week, all the pre-cancers will turn red; skin can become very irritated and crusty. Heals 1 week after finishing treatment.

Less irritating but slower treatment than Efudex®. Similar reaction.

Area may become irritated. Amount of irritation varies from mild to severe, depending on patient. Heals 1 week after complete treatment.

Slowest and least irritating of the creams. Can only be used for actinic keratoses.

May cause redness, swelling, peeling, and crusting. Important to avoid sunlight and bright light sources for 2 days after treatment.

Depending on size and location, it may take about 1 month for open wound to heal. Apply Vaseline and bandages daily until completely healed.

Sutures are removed in 1–3 weeks. Strength of wound at 2 weeks is only 5 percent so avoid heavy lifting and pulling on the skin for one month.

Sutures are removed in 1–2 weeks. Recovery similar to that for excision. End scar will be longer because of the amount of tissue removed.

Expect a smaller scar since only tissue containing cancer will be removed. This type of surgery is appropriate for high-risk sites, and sites next to vital structures like the eye, nose, or mouth.

Radiation is delivered daily 3–5 times per week for several weeks. Treated skin is essentially burned and can develop a wound, healing 2 weeks after complete treatment.

See doctor 3 times a week for injections, for 3 weeks. No downtime.

Fatigue and flu-like symptoms are common after each dose. Usually inject interferon 3 times a week for 1 year.

# Treatment for skin cancers

SKIN CANCERS CAN BE TREATED IN A VARIETY OF WAYS. THE BEST METHOD AND CURE RATES CAN BE DISCUSSED WITH YOUR DOCTOR. It will depend on the type of cancer, location, size, and your preference.

Treatment methods include creams, photodynamic therapy, a "scrape and burn" procedure, excision, Mohs surgery, and radiation. Treatment for melanoma most commonly involves excision. If your melanoma is deep, you may be given the option to have sentinel lymph node biopsy, lymph node dissection, radiation, chemotherapy, interferon, or other experimental therapy.

# What is Mohs surgery?

Mohs surgery was named after Frederick Mohs, MD. It is a tissue sparing technique for removing skin cancer. Only highly credentialed physicians with specific training are considered Mohs surgeons.

Mohs surgery is important because tumors do not grow as spheres or circles. They follow paths of least resistance and frequently have long arms or tentacles. Though you see a round papule, the tumor cells may actually be shaped very irregularly and much of the tumor may be invisible to the naked eye. Mohs surgery removes the tumor, sparing normal tissue.

Using local anesthesia, the area around the skin cancer is numbed. The excised tissue is like a piecrust, and the pie is cut horizontally. The surgeon performing the surgery also checks the tumor under the microscope. The color maps are used to determine exactly where the tumor's tentacles begin and end. If cancer is seen at any edge of the "piecrust," then more tumor is cut out. The Mohs surgeon goes back and forth between the skin cancer and the microscope, until the entire tumor is removed. Once the periphery is clear, then patients are brought back to the procedure room for stitching to repair the wound.

If you are scheduled for Mohs surgery, keep in mind that your surgeon cannot predict if all the cancer will be removed during the first stage, or if multiple stages will be needed. Each time tissue is excised, it takes approximately one hour to process and look at it under the microscope. Plan ahead to bring a book or snack.

## Did you know?

▸ Excision removes the cancer 95 percent of the time. Mohs surgery offers a 99 percent cure rate.

▸ You can put cream anesthetic on an hour before your surgery. This will make the numbing injections less painful.

▸ The dermatologist performing Mohs surgery should be "fellowship-trained." This means they spent an extra year formally learning this technique. For more information please visit www.mohscollege.com.

# If it's not a skin cancer, what else could it be?

OBVIOUSLY NOT EVERY BUMP OR DISCOLORATION ON THE SKIN IS A CANCER. It takes years to learn how to tell the difference between a brown bump that is a benign lesion or melanoma. So it's important to ask your dermatologist if you're not sure. Here is a list of common skin lesions, discussed further in the chapter on general dermatology.

| Common benign skin conditions | Things to worry about |
| --- | --- |
| Freckles | Actinic keratosis (pre-cancer) |
| Lentigo (LIVER SPOT) | Lentigo maligna |
| Telangiectasia (TINY VEIN) | Basal cell carcinoma |
| Hemangioma | Basel cell carcinoma, melanoma |
| Wart | Squamous cell carcinoma |
| Psoriasis | Squamous cell carcinoma |
| Seborrheic keratosis (BROWN, WAXY SPOT) | Melanoma |
| Skin-colored bump | Basal cell carcinoma |
| Regular moles | Melanoma |

It's very important to familiarize yourself with your skin so you can spot changes. A board-certified dermatologist should evaluate changing moles and new moles. A dermatologist studies patterns and easily sees over 200,000 moles during training, so he or she can usually can tell if a lesion is benign or malignant just by looking. Of course, there are some lesions that are borderline and difficult to interpret. These should be biopsied and looked at under the microscope.

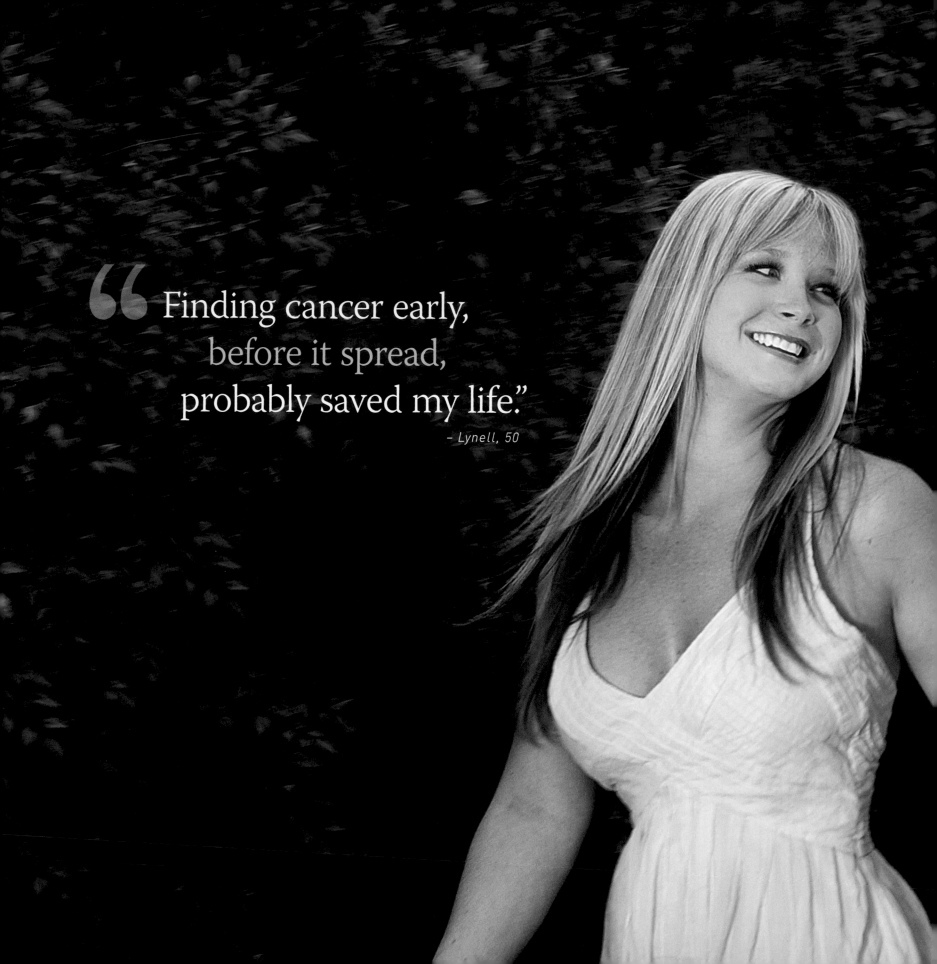

" Finding cancer early, before it spread, probably saved my life."

– Lynell, 50

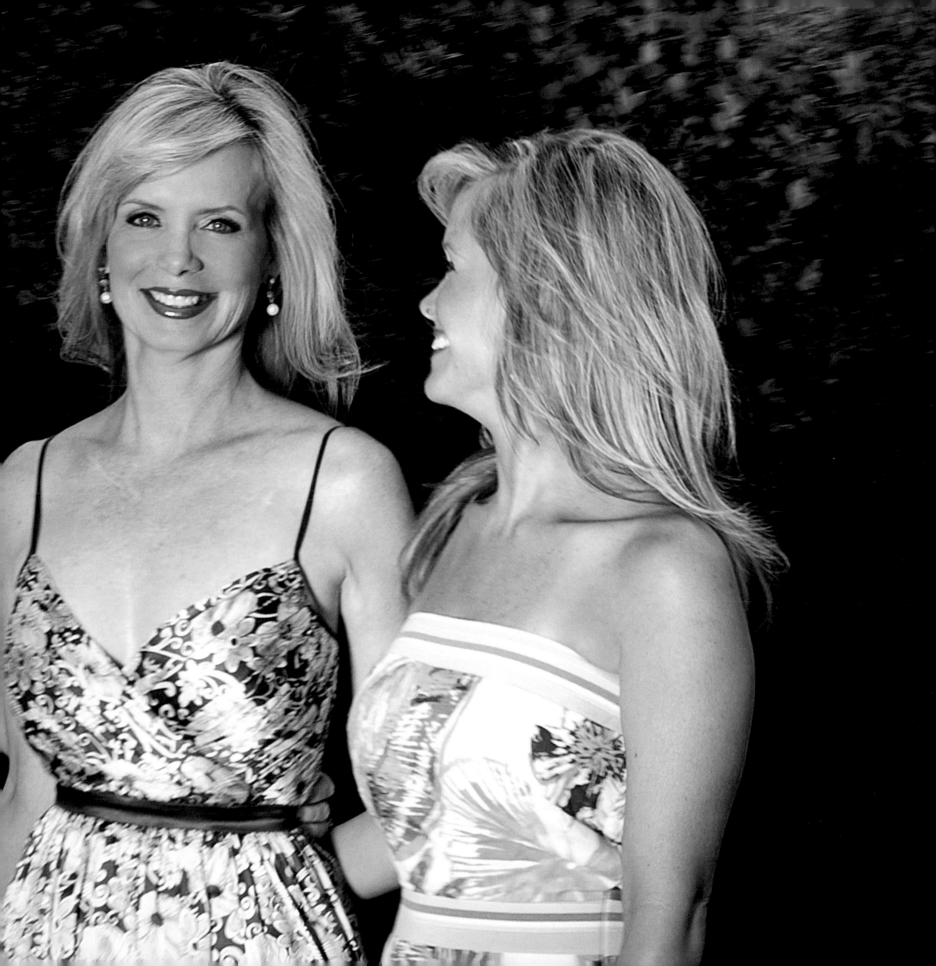

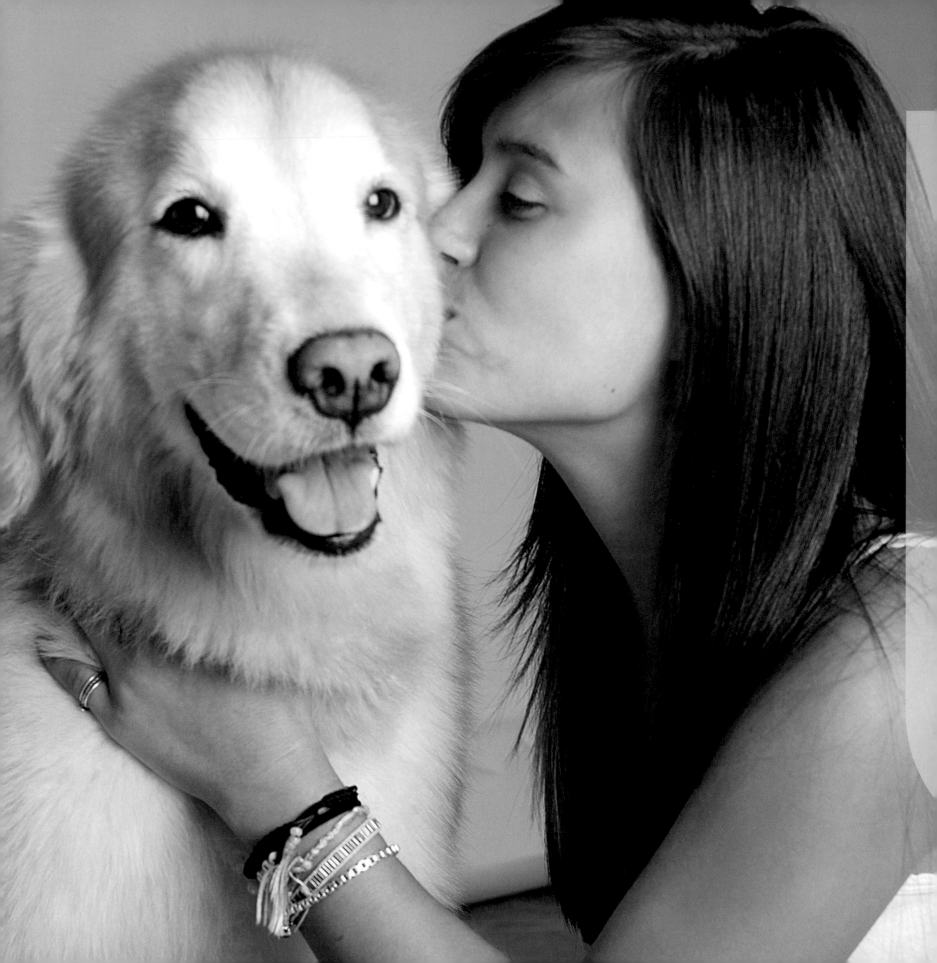

# CHAPTER 9

# SCARS & STRETCH MARKS

> ❝ **Almost eight years ago,** my dog, Shasta, attacked and bit me along the chin.
>
> **I NEEDED TWO RECONSTRUCTIVE SURGERIES.**❞
>
> – *Kiana, 15*

Scars and stretch marks are constant reminders of the past that can stand in the way of smooth, beautiful skin—but there is hope. Scar appearance can be improved by many therapies—from creams to dressings to injections. The appropriate therapy will depend on the particular scar type. Laser therapy, a newer modality, has shown promising results in diminishing scar redness, texture, and appearance.

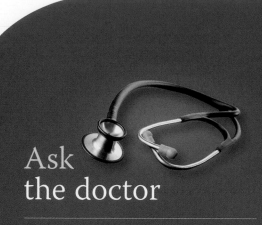

## Ask the doctor

**IS THERE A MAGIC CREAM THAT CAN ERASE SCARS?**

No, there is no cream scientifically proven to erase scars. Some creams show minimal improvement, perhaps because they require massage. Some surgeons recommend massaging the wound after surgery to reduce swelling and scar prominence, but only after the skin edges are well healed. Ask your surgeon when it's safe to start massaging.

**WHAT CAN I DO TO IMPROVE MY SCARS?**

In the past, surgery was the only way to improve scars. The unsightly or bumpy scar is excised by a dermatologic surgeon or plastic surgeon, and then the new wound is resutured carefully. This results in a fine line scar in most cases.

Today, lasers can improve redness, texture, and overall appearance of the scar.

## Why it occurs

Every time the skin is injured or cut, cells are recruited to stop bleeding and clean the wound. Cells and chemicals are released to stimulate growth of blood vessels and collagen to make new skin.

If a prolonged or overzealous healing response occurs, a hypertrophic scar or keloid may develop.

A **HYPERTROPHIC SCAR** is raised above the original wound. Hypertrophic scars can occur on any part of the body.

A **KELOID** is not only raised, but also spreads beyond the boundaries of the original wound. This usually occurs in darker-skinned patients. Common locations for keloids include the ears after piercing, the central chest, and the upper shoulders. There may be a familial predisposition to keloid formation.

Scar formation may occur after any injury. The best dermatologic and plastic surgeons use refined and meticulous stitching techniques to create barely visible scars.

The wound healing process continues for months, so your scar will gradually improve over the first six months to a year.

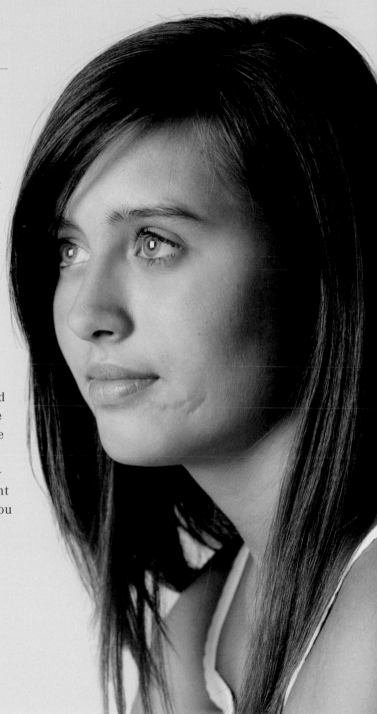

# " Kiana's story

Almost eight years ago, my dog, Shasta, attacked me. I was bitten along the chin and needed two reconstructive surgeries. I loved my dog, though she put me through a lot of psychological and physical pain. I was in counseling for the first year, and it was very difficult for me to talk about it because I was so young. Everyone would ask me, 'What happened?' One parent even said, 'You have chocolate sauce on your face.'

I have had multiple laser treatments since age 7 to help with the scars. My pediatrician prescribed Xanax®, which helped me relax before and during the procedure. The laser felt like a rubber band snapping against my skin.

I have been through a lot in the past 15 years, so here is my advice: Always bring something to read or keep you busy. Bring an iPod so you don't have to hear the laser. After a while you get used to the bruising that happens after laser treatment. Your scar will turn red/blue. Do not forget to wear sunscreen. I have darker skin, and it is very important that I wear sunscreen or it will turn dark. Also, you can't get laser treatment if you are too tan.

The laser has helped me a lot, even though the scars will always be a part of me."

AGE: 15
CONCERN: SCAR
TREATMENT: VBEAM LASER
NUMBER OF TREATMENTS: 10
DOWNTIME: 3-5 DAYS
BRUISING

BEFORE

AFTER

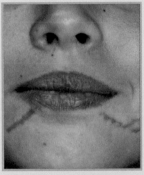

# Treatment options

Treatment options for scars include intralesional injections of steroids or 5-fluorouracil, pulsed-dye laser treatment and fractionated laser treatment. Radiation, cryotherapy, interferon, and silicone gel sheets or other dressings have also been used.

**INTRALESIONAL STEROIDS** soften and flatten hypertrophic scars and keloids. To see noticeable improvement, monthly injections are often necessary. Injections can be diluted with lidocaine to decrease discomfort. Potential side effects include pain with injection, atrophy, telangiectasias, and hypopigmentation.

**5-FLUOROURACIL** (5-FU) is believed to reduce postoperative scarring by decreasing collagen proliferation. Injections, which are typically combined with intralesional steroids, are given monthly. The solution is injected into the center of the scar tissue until a slight blanching (whitening) is observed. Multiple injections separated by approximately 1 cm may be needed. Only the raised portions of the scar are injected.

**PULSED-DYE LASER** not only reduces redness, but also height, blending the scar with surrounding skin. Early intervention with pulsed-dye laser therapy may control the extent of new blood vessel growth within the wound and prevent scar formation. Treatments are performed every four to eight weeks. 5-FU and intralesional steroid injections may be given simultaneously. See Chapter 4 for details on how this laser works.

**FRACTIONATED LASER SYSTEMS** can reduce height and improve overall appearance of scars after surgery, burns, or trauma. These lasers are unique because they can be used for hypertrophic (raised) or atrophic (depressed) scars. See Chapter 6 for details on how fractionated lasers work. Laser treatment of scars, even scars resulting from a medically necessary procedure, is usually not covered by insurance.

**SILICONE GEL SHEET** or a dressing, such as Ultrathin Duoderm®, can be a useful adjunct in the prevention and/or treatment of scars.

A multifaceted approach to treatment of hypertrophic scars and keloids may include 5-FU to suppress collagen formation, corticosteroids to suppress inflammation, and pulsed-dye laser to suppress blood vessel formation.

# Mary's story

A few years ago, I decided to have a facelift, brow lift, and a chemical peel around my mouth. Everything that could go wrong did. I was allergic to the adhesive tape, resulting in raw wounds from my ears onto my cheeks. After the chemical peel, I developed herpes blisters around my lips. The pain and scarring were horrible. I could barely open my mouth. I literally gave up and thought I would remain like that for the rest of my life.

Then in January 2005, I went to a neurosurgeon about my back, and he immediately (before we even talked about my back pain) told me to get to a GOOD dermatologist to see about my face. For the first few laser treatments, a nurse had to hold my mouth open so I could be numbed. I went in once a month for a year for laser treatments and cortisone shots.

The results have been totally amazing. With a little makeup, the scars hardly show at all. Most importantly, I feel good about how I've come out of this horrible experience. When I was asked for permission to show my pictures and tell my story, I gave it enthusiastically. I hope it will help someone else get through a hard time."

AGE: 77
CONCERN: SCAR
TREATMENT: VBEAM LASER
NUMBER OF TREATMENTS: 9
DOWNTIME: 3–5 DAYS
BRUISING

BEFORE

AFTER

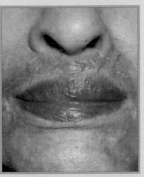

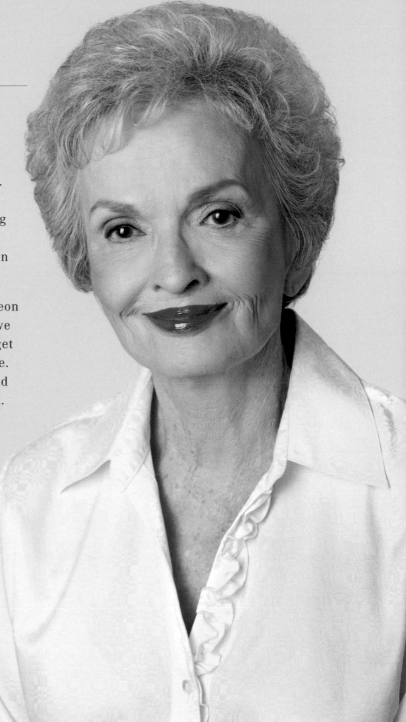

# Stretch marks: my story

I was 13 when I started noticing stretch marks on my inner thighs. They were bright red, and I was very self-conscious about them. It was spring, and I wanted to be able to wear shorts and swimsuits like all of my friends did. So I went to my physician, and we tried some topical treatments, but they didn't work.

I was referred to a dermatologist who took one look at the marks and said, 'I can fix that.' I started with two Vbeam® treatments and then had five Fraxel® treatments over the course of about 10 months. I was sore and red for only about two to four days after each treatment, but each time it got easier and the recovery was faster. With each treatment I saw improvement and was very excited the marks were fading away. A lot of my friends and family have noticed great improvement also.

Since my treatment, I have been able to wear shorts and swimsuits without having to worry about people staring at my legs. I am also a dancer, and we always have to wear shorts and costumes. Now my legs won't distract me or anyone else from my performance."

AGE: 14
CONCERN: STRETCH MARKS
TREATMENT: VBEAM LASER AND
FRAXEL RE:STORE LASER
NUMBER OF TREATMENTS:
2 VBEAM, 5 FRAXEL
DOWNTIME: 3–4 DAYS
REDNESS AND SWELLING

BEFORE

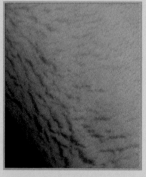

AFTER

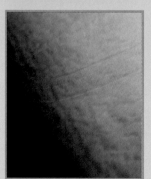

# Why it occurs

Stretch marks are difficult to treat. We do not know why some people develop them, yet others do not.

Stretch marks tend to appear after rapid growth. They are common around the biceps of men who lift weights, around the breasts and hips of young women during puberty, and on the abdomen of women after pregnancy. They can also occur with rapid weight loss or in those taking anabolic steroids. There may be a genetic predisposition for the development of stretch marks.

**STRIAE RUBRA** – When stretch marks first appear, they tend to be red or purplish. These are called striae rubra. The redness can be reduced with a pulsed-dye laser, and this is satisfactory for most patients.

**STRIAE DISTENSAE** – Even without laser treatment, most stretch marks later lose their red color and become dark or white wrinkled streaks. These are called striae distensae. Studies suggest these stretch marks may benefit from non-ablative lasers.

# Treatment options

Treatment options for stretch marks include topical agents such as tretinoin (Retin-A®), ascorbic acid (vitamin C) and glycolic acid. A limited number of effective treatments are available for striae rubra. However, the pulsed-dye laser has been found to produce moderate results.

Fractionated lasers have been reported to diminish the appearance of stretch marks. It may improve them by stimulating collagen and elastic fiber remodeling or synthesis. This fills the wrinkled stretch marks resulting in a smoother appearance. Cost is based on extent of the areas to be treated and number of treatments needed.

**PATIENT T!P**

Although cocoa butter and vitamin E have been used as moisturizing agents, there is little clinical evidence to support their use in the prevention or treatment of stretch marks.

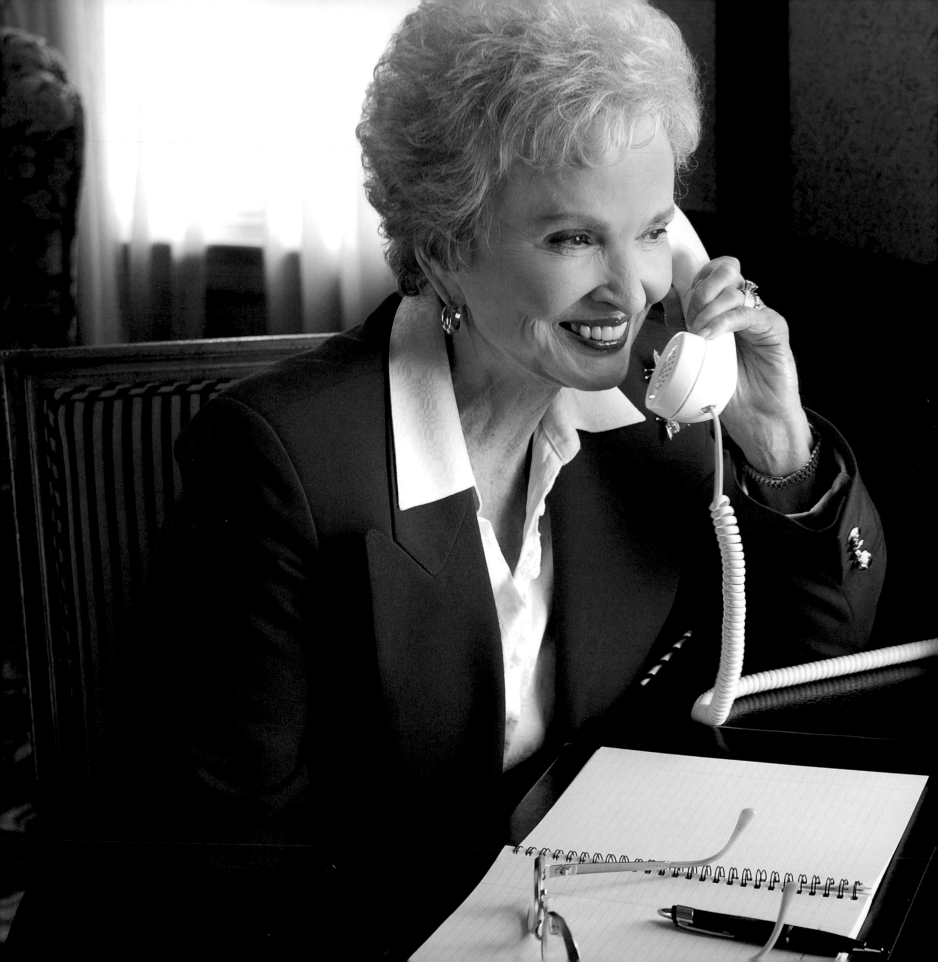

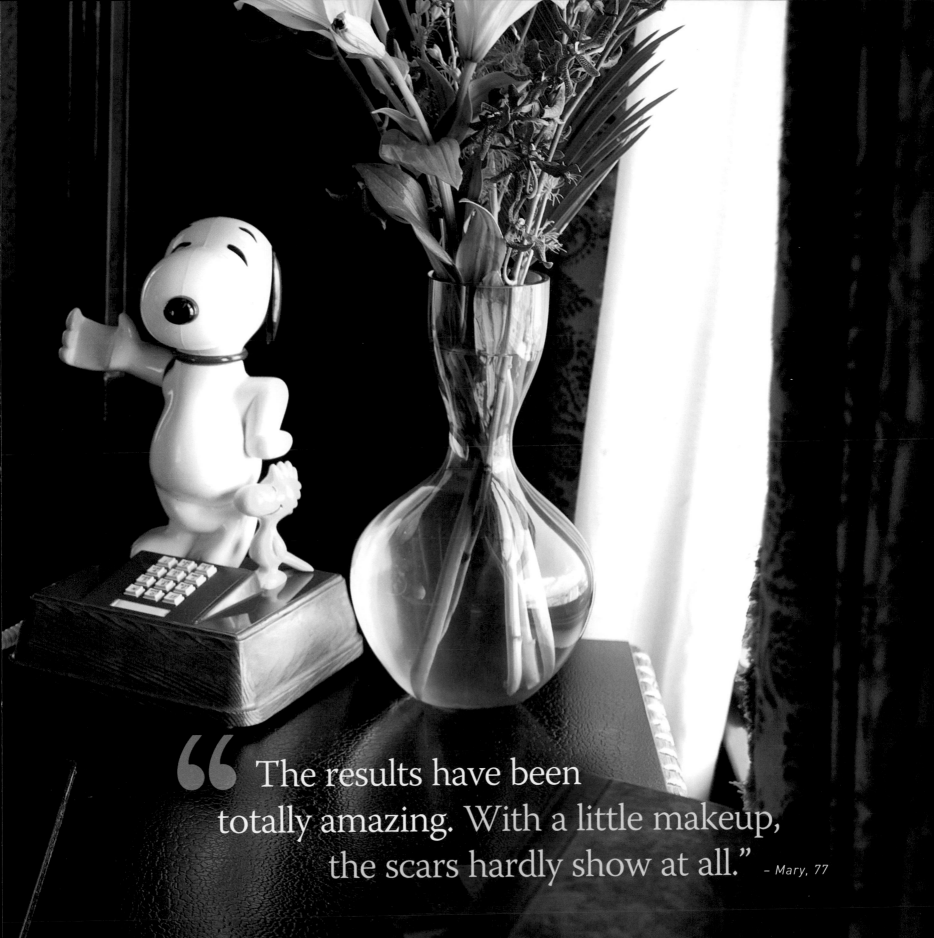

" The results have been
totally amazing. With a little makeup,
the scars hardly show at all." – Mary, 77

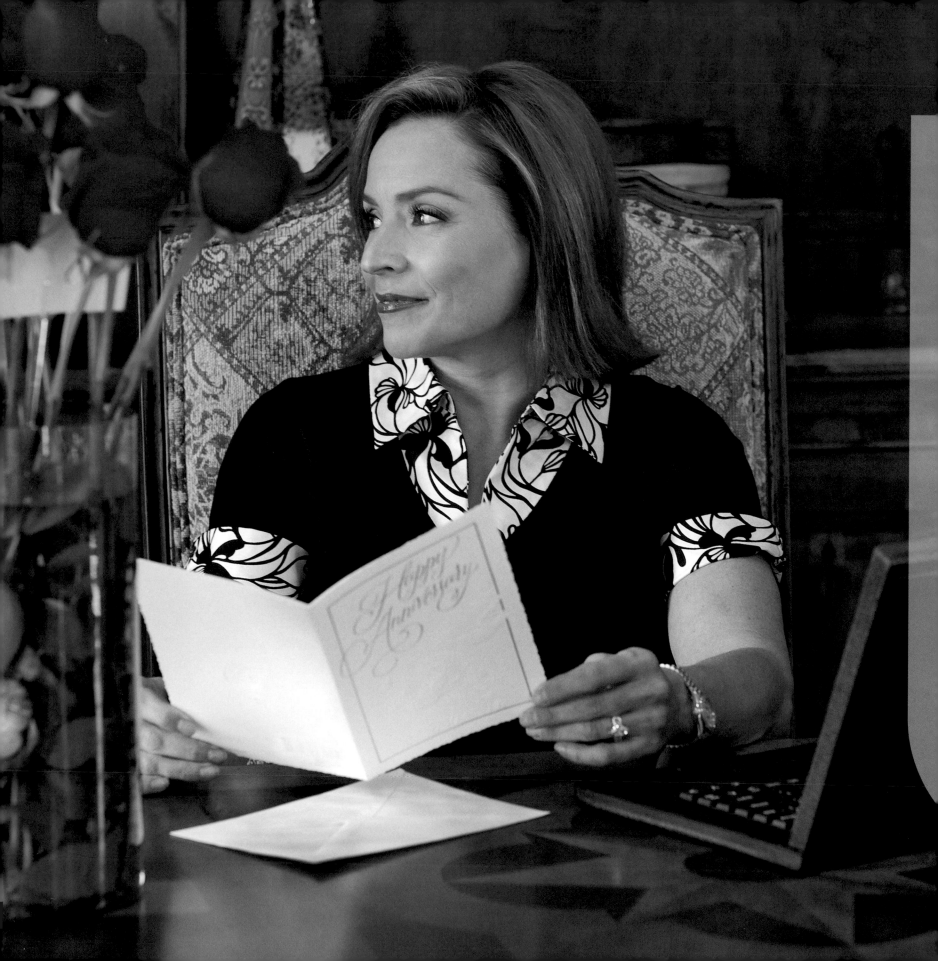

# CHAPTER 10

# GENERAL DERM

## "It was depressing every time I looked in the mirror, AND NOTHING SEEMED TO HELP."

*– Samie, 50*

Obviously, not every bump or discoloration on the skin is a cancer. This chapter covers the most common skin bumps, rashes and conditions. It takes years to learn how to tell the difference between a spot that is harmless and a dangerous skin cancer. So ask your dermatologist. But when he or she tells you the long name of your condition, the information here can help you decode it.

# What it is, why it occurs

 **FRECKLES** — Freckles are brown spots on the skin that appear during early childhood. Found on sun-exposed areas (face, outer arms) of people with light skin, they may be inherited. While they don't become melanomas, freckles are markers of sun damage in fair patients, so they indicate patients at risk for developing melanomas. Freckles darken with sun exposure and lighten with the use of sunblock or during the winter.

 **SOLAR LENTIGINES (LIVER SPOTS)** — Lentigines look similar to freckles. They are flat brown spots on sun-exposed skin. They are the result of chronic sun exposure, so they appear during adulthood. They may fade a little with sun avoidance and age but usually do not go away. Solar lentigines are benign.

 **MELASMA (MASK OF PREGNANCY)** — Dark brown patches on the forehead, cheeks, around the nose, or the upper lip may be melasma. It can be caused or exacerbated by pregnancy, oral contraceptives, and sun exposure. Melasma is discussed further in Chapter 1.

 **TELANGIECTASIA (SPIDER VEINS)** — These tiny dilated blood vessels on the skin look like a red line or group of red lines (spider veins). If just one or two are present, they are probably related to fair skin and sun exposure. If there are many, then other diagnoses should be considered, including rosacea. See rosacea in Chapter 4.

 **CHERRY HEMANGIOMA** — A small red or purple bump made up of a group of blood vessels is called a cherry hemangioma. These are common on the chest and back. Most people over age 60 have at least one or two, and some patients have many more.

 **ANGIOFIBROMA** — This skin-colored bump develops during adulthood, usually on the nose. It is comprised of blood vessels and fibrous tissue.

 **REGULAR MOLES** — There are three kinds of regular moles. Junctional moles are flat and brown. Compound moles are raised and brown. Intradermal moles are raised and skin-colored. Regular moles often start out flat and brown during childhood, then become raised and lose some of their color during early adulthood. This particular change is normal, but a dermatologist should evaluate any changing mole.

# Samie's story

My appearance is important to me, and I plan to age as gracefully as possible. I'm 50 years old and the mother of two grown sons. Also, I just became a grandmother, and I'm looking forward to that part of my life. We're a very close family and spend a lot of time together. Also, I enjoy cooking, reading and traveling.

I never had skin problems until I began to get large brown spots on my face about two years ago. It was depressing every time I looked in the mirror, and nothing seemed to help.

I tried microdermabrasion, but it didn't have any effect. Then I visited a laser specialist, who told me I had melasma and suggested Fraxel laser treatments.

I'm so glad he did! I had five treatments, one each month. After three treatments, I saw amazing results. Each time I had a treatment I had a little redness and slight swelling, and I always stayed at home for a couple of days afterwards to rest my face. The pain wasn't intense, but if you're going to have a laser treatment you need to know there will be a burning sensation during and after the procedure. I have found it's really important to sleep with your head propped up on a couple of pillows the first night after treatment.

My family and friends have noticed the change in my skin, and that makes it all worth it. They say it has a glow, and they're right. I'm proud of my appearance again."

AGE: 50
CONCERN: MELASMA
TREATMENT:
FRAXEL RE:STORE LASER
NUMBER OF TREATMENTS: 5
DOWNTIME: 2 DAYS SWELLING
AND REDNESS

BEFORE

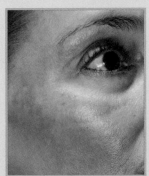

AFTER

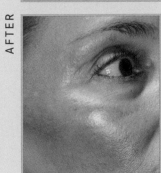

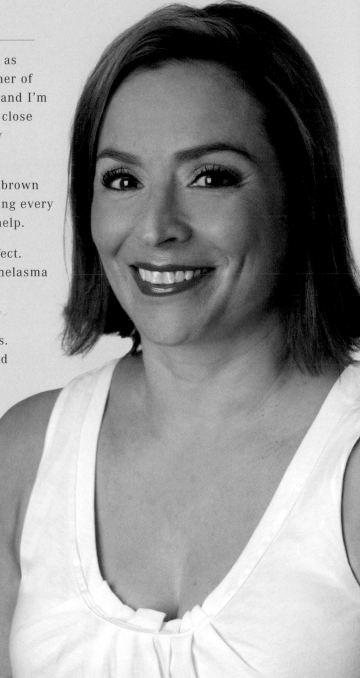

# What it is, why it occurs (continued)

 **DERMATOFIBROMA** — A firm, tan, pink or brown bump, dermatofibroma is frequently mistaken for a mole. They are a special type of scar that is formed after an insect bite or other trauma. They are commonly found on arms and legs.

 **SEBORRHEIC KERATOSIS** — These waxy yellow or brown bumps can appear anywhere — face, chest, back, arms, and legs. There is a flat version too. They begin to appear after age 40 and are very common. They can become itchy or irritated, especially if they catch on clothing.

 **SEBACEOUS HYPERPLASIA** — A yellow bump on the face, which represents an overgrown oil gland. Sebaceous hyperplasia can occur with rosacea. This is further discussed in Chapter 4.

 **KERATOSIS PILARIS** — Tiny bumps, like little spines, are felt on the back of the upper arms or upper thighs. This is a chronic condition caused by plugged skin over each hair follicle.

 **ACNE** — Hair follicle occlusion, bacteria, and oil secretion lead to the comedone (whitehead or blackhead). Disruption of the hair follicle and inflammation turn the comedone into a pimple, pustule or cyst. For more information on acne, see Chapter 2.

 **EPIDERMOID CYST** — A bump under the skin with a central pore, an epidermoid cyst is filled with keratin. Patients frequently squeeze out white material to flatten, only to have the cyst refill. When irritated, epidermoid cysts can become red and tender. They can occur anywhere, including the scalp or back. Treatment is steroid injections or excision.

 **MILIA** — This is just a tiny cyst, usually 1-2 mm and often on the face or scalp.

**WARTS** — Caused by the human papillomavirus (HPV), the common wart is frequently on the hand or foot. It is a skin-colored bump with a warty surface. The virus stimulates skin growth and new vessel formation; tiny black dots inside the wart represent clogged blood vessels. The virus hides inside your skin cell so your immune system cannot see it. There are many treatment options: over-the-counter salicylic acid, duct tape, freezing, and injections. Multiple treatments will be needed. You may need to see a dermatologist for stubborn lesions.

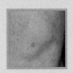

**LIPOMA** — Soft bumps or lumps of fat under the skin, lipomas range from golf ball to kitchen sponge size. Although it is not certain why they form, they are benign and do not need to be treated. If there are many blood vessels inside the lipoma it can be painful. All lumps under the skin should be examined by a doctor to exclude cancer.

**DRY SKIN OR XEROSIS** — Often, when patients complain of itchy skin they really have dry skin, which occurs when your skin doesn't make enough lipids. The best moisturizers contain ingredients to help lipids penetrate and humectants to retain water. The best time to moisturize is immediately after a bath or shower. See Chapter 10 on skin products.

**BRUISES** — Bruising on the forearms and hands in older individuals can be secondary to minimal trauma resulting from a loss of collagen over years of sun damage. The medical term is solar purpura. This condition is aggravated by blood thinners such as aspirin or coumadin.

**LEATHERY SKIN OR DERMATOHELIOSIS** — Over time, sun and aging lead to changes in the skin, such as thickening and discoloration. Dermatoheliosis is the technical term for photodamage. See Chapter 1 for causes and treatment options.

**SEBORRHEIC DERMATITIS OR DANDRUFF** — Dandruff can occur not only on the scalp, but also on the face and around the ears. On the face, it looks like pink scaly patches in and between the eyebrows, in the creases of your nose, around your mouth, and inside or behind the ears. Men frequently get it in their beard or on the chest. Seborrheic dermatitis is caused by yeast that live in the follicle. One solution is to apply a dandruff shampoo to the scalp and/or other affected areas for 15 minutes and then rinse off. Another option is an over-the-counter mild steroid to help the redness.

# What it is, why it occurs (continued)

 **ALLERGIC DERMATITIS** — This refers to either contact or irritant allergy. Patients can be allergic to rubber, hair dye, preservatives, or a myriad of substances. Exposure causes an allergic contact dermatitis. For example, exposure to poison ivy causes a bright red and weepy rash with tiny clear blisters. Repeated exposure to an allergen, such as rubber gloves in a sensitized individual, can cause a dry, itchy rash, similar to eczema. To determine if you have a contact allergy, a dermatologist may apply patches with various allergens to your back. This is not the same as an allergist injecting tiny amounts of allergens to your back or arm, which tests for systemic allergies.

 **ECZEMA** — Eczema is a term synonymous with "dermatitis." This refers to a rash, which is red, dry, and usually itchy. Atopic dermatitis is a subtype of eczema classically seen in children on the cheeks, elbows, and the backs of the knees.

 **PSORIASIS** — These uniquely red areas of skin covered with silvery thick scale commonly occur on the elbows, knees, and scalp. There may be a genetic component in a subset of patients. Psoriasis is thought to be an immune-mediated inflammatory disease of the skin. Many exciting new treatment options are available for this condition, so please see your doctor.

 **HAIR LOSS** — The two main causes for hair loss are stress and genetics. Stress, such as giving birth, undergoing surgery, or psychological stress can cause the hair to fall out diffusely within three months of the acute stressor. In this case, the hair will grow back, but the new growth may not be noticeable for months. Genetics and hormones cause the hair to fall out slowly, mainly from the front and top of the scalp. Rogaine® topical solution or foam may help slow hair loss by stimulating hair growth.

 **EXCESS HAIR** — Hairs on the upper lip, chin, or sides of the face in females can be a sign of excess male hormone, and you should see your dermatologist or endocrinologist for possible laboratory evaluation. Many hair removal options exist; please refer to the treatment section of this chapter.

**BRITTLE NAILS** — Many factors contribute to brittle nails including normal aging, a lack of moisture, dry heat, nail polish remover and harsh chemicals. Certain nail polishes and nail hardeners can also play a role in brittle nails. Medical conditions which may play a role include thyroid disease, vitamin deficiency, and anemia.

# Treatment comments

The treatment of **pigmented lesions**, including hair and tattoos, is similar, usually with a laser that targets pigment. This is discussed in Chapter 1.

**Vascular lesions**, like telangiectasias and hemangiomas, can be treated with lasers. This is covered in Chapters 4 and 5.

**Angiofibromas, moles, dermatofibromas, and seborrheic keratoses** are benign, but they can be removed if bothersome.

Sebaceous hyperplasia, milia, keratosis pilaris, acne, and cysts have multiple treatment options that range from creams to procedures. Milia can be treated with extraction. Keratosis pilaris can be treated with urea or lactic acid cream. Acne usually involves multiple treatments to help current lesions and prevent the formation of new lesions. Acne is one the most treatable skin conditions; seek a physician before you develop scars.

**Warts** can be resistant to treatment, but there are many options. If over-the-counter salicylic acid does not work, or if you have multiple warts, your doctor can help. Common therapies include paring, freezing with liquid nitrogen, or an immune-stimulator cream called Aldara®. Some dermatologists also perform injections.

**Lipomas** are benign but can be surgically removed.

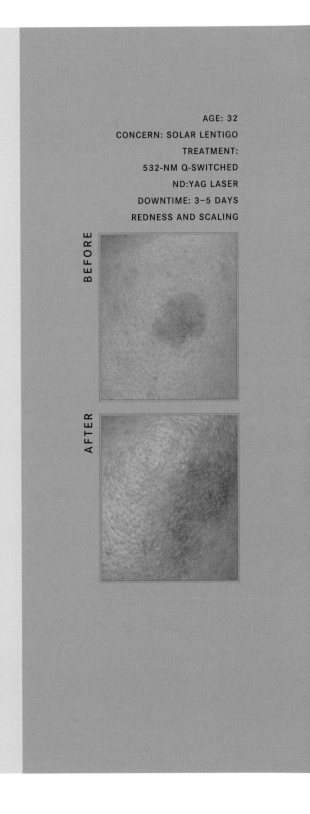

AGE: 32
CONCERN: SOLAR LENTIGO
TREATMENT:
532-NM Q-SWITCHED
ND:YAG LASER
DOWNTIME: 3–5 DAYS
REDNESS AND SCALING

BEFORE

AFTER

# Treatment comments (continued)

**Dry skin** is treated with moisturizers. See skin care product discussion in Chapter 10.

**Bruises** can be difficult to treat. Arnica is an herbal topical that may help bruises resolve more quickly. Tretinoin cream applied to the forearms and hands can stimulate collagen production and diminish bruising. Vitamin K has been shown to reduce bruising after laser procedures, but it does not necessarily improve incidental bruising on fragile skin. Recently, the pulsed-dye laser has been shown to expedite the resolution of bruising.

**Leathery skin**, or **dermatoheliosis**, can be improved in multiple ways, depending on how aggressive you want to be. Read Chapter 3 for more information about photoaging and wrinkles.

**Dermatitis, seborrheic dermatitis, allergic dermatitis, eczema, and psoriasis** are all common dermatologic problems with multiple treatment options. Please see a general dermatologist to discuss the right treatment for you.

Temporary **hair removal** options include shaving, waxing, threading, plucking, and epilating. It is a myth that following these treaments, more hairs grow back or that hairs grow back thicker. A prescription cream called Vaniqa® slows hair growth, so hair removal sessions can be less frequent. Laser hair removal has been shown to effectively reduce hair density, but several treatments are required, often spaced four to six weeks apart.

**Brittle nails** can be treated by limiting contact with harsh chemicals, nail polishes, and nail polish removers. A visit with your general medical doctor may be warranted to exclude thyroid abnormalities, vitamin deficiencies, or anemia. Conditioning the nails and cuticles with a gentle moisturizer may provide some benefit. Biotin supplements can strengthen the nails as well.

## PATIENT T!P

A note on retinoids and hair removal: stop your retinoid cream one or even two weeks before waxing to prevent the wax from removing skin.

# Treatment of pigmented lesions, tattoos and hair

AGE: 23

CONCERN: PROFESSIONAL
TATTOO REMOVAL

TREATMENT: 1064-NM
Q-SWITCHED ND: YAG LASER

NUMBER OF TREATMENTS: 13

DOWNTIME: 3–5 DAYS

MINIMAL REDNESS, SWELLING,
AND CRUSTING

TO REITERATE, FRECKLES, LENTIGINES, AND MELASMA ARE BENIGN (HARMLESS). If they are located on the face or especially bothersome, they can be treated with freezing, cauterizing, or a laser that targets pigment, such as the Q-switched Nd:YAG, alexandrite, or ruby laser. Fractionated lasers have also been effective.

Tattoos are made up of pigment, so are treated with similar lasers. Q-switched lasers are designed to put all of the laser's energy into a short burst. This powerful burst of energy perfectly targets the tiny pigment particles. Most tattoo colors can be significantly lightened with multiple treatments; between five and 10 treatments may be needed. Red, skin-colored, and white tattoo ink can turn black with Q-switched lasers, so these pigments should be removed instead with ablative lasers such as the carbon dioxide or erbium:YAG laser. It is imperative to seek an experienced physician for tattoo removal.

Hair also contains a lot of pigment, and this is the target when using lasers to remove hair. The colored hair becomes hot and transfers heat to the surrounding follicle. The follicle is heated and destroyed. Immediately after the laser procedure, the hair easily falls out. Because only a third of hair follicles are in the growing stage, only one third of hairs can be treated at each session. After treatment, hairs from other stages will grow in, which is completely normal.

Because the target is pigment within the hair shaft, the best candidates for laser hair removal have fair skin and dark hair. Darker skin patients have pigment in their skin, and the laser will heat both the pigment in the skin and the pigment in the hair. Heating the skin can lead to hyperpigmentation, and in some cases burns. Darker skin patients can still be treated; however, they should see an experienced physician. Also, a longer wavelength laser, such as the 1064-nm long-pulsed Nd:YAG, should be used.

BEFORE

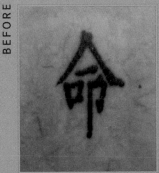

AFTER

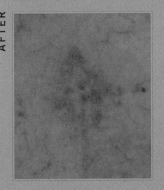

## Did you know?

A new generation of permanent tattoo ink called infinitink™ is made of compounds designed to be safe for the skin and easier to remove compared to conventional tattoo ink. For more information visit www.infinitink.com.

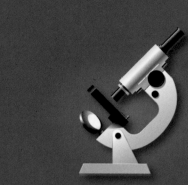

# The science
## revealed

HOME LASER HAIR REMOVAL TREATMENTS HAVE BECOME A POPULAR WAY TO REMOVE UNWANTED HAIR GROWTH. An example is the TRIA Personal Laser Hair Removal System, the first laser hair removal system cleared by the FDA for home use.

The TRIA system was developed by the scientists who invented the first professional diode laser hair removal systems in 1993. Since then, this group has found a way to miniaturize the technology and make it safe for home use. An appropriate user of this technology is defined as an individual with naturally light brown to black hair in the treatment area and lighter skin type, excluding darker skinned individuals. A 40 percent hair reduction has been reported six months after three treatments.

The Silk'n, a novel low-energy pulsed-light device for home-use hair removal, is marketed by Home Skinovations. It has been shown to reduce hair counts by 38 percent to 54 percent with the lower legs exhibiting greater hair reduction than arms, groin and underarm.

# What to expect
## (time, cost, recovery, permanence, risk)

NUMBING IS NOT USUALLY NECESSARY BUT CAN BE USED. If you are treating hair, the hair may be shaved immediately before treatment.

Each pulse of the laser will feel like a tiny burst of heat. The laser will target the birthmark, hairy area, or tattoo, leaving a gray crust over the skin. You'll hear a pitter patter sequence of bursts in a row. If you are treating hair, you may be able to smell burning hair. If your tattoo has different colors, you may need to use different lasers.

Immediately after treatment you'll see the superficial crust of heated skin on the surface. Just apply Vaseline® daily and keep the area moist and covered. This will allow the crust to be replaced by new skin without scabbing. You should be healed in a week or two. Return monthly for the next treatment.

Most pigmented lesions (including hair and tattoos) will need to be treated multiple times. The number of treatments will depend on the condition.

Again, only the hairs in the growing stage can be treated. Soon after treatment, hairs in the resting cycle may start to grow. These hairs were not treated by the laser and it is normal for hairs to grow back. Several treatments, perhaps three to five, will be needed to treat all the hairs.

Treatment time may vary based on the areas treated; plan on 10-30 minutes. Cost may be per area or per pulse.

# " Nancy's story

I remember the first time my mother let me shave my legs. I was so excited when she handed me a bar of soap and a disposable pink plastic razor, and I paid close attention as she revealed the secret to smooth, silky-soft legs. But before long, shaving became a chore.

I liked the long-lasting smoothness waxing delivered, but I didn't like waiting between appointments. Then I tried laser hair removal in a doctor's office, which I found excruciatingly painful. I developed blisters and dark spots, and the doctor (not a dermatologist) said I shouldn't continue the treatment.

After my skin healed, I used bleaching crèmes to remove the dark spots the laser had lifted in my skin. I went back to shaving and decided that razor bumps were better than blisters.

Shaving alternatives did not cross my mind until I received the Tria hair-removal system as a gift. It's virtually impossible to develop a burn or darkening of the skin with Tria if it is used on the correct skin type.

I use my Tria once a month; I test, shave and then treat the area. I have treated my legs, underarms and bikini area four times in the past four months, and I am amazed with the results. I shave once a week and stay smooth the entire time. And it's virtually painless."

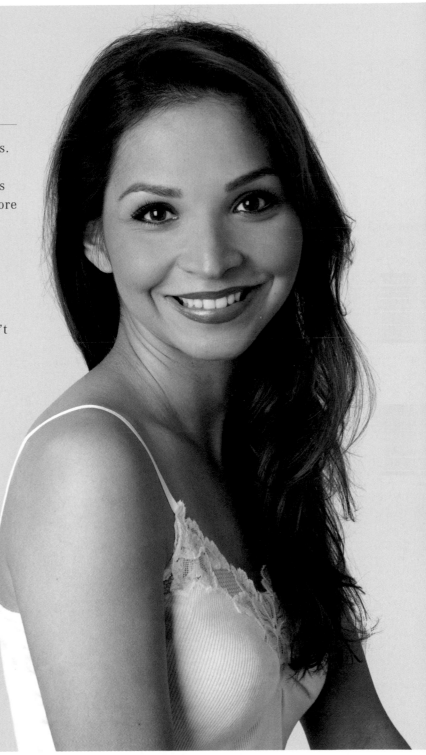

"I am amazed with the results
and how smooth my skin feels."

– Nancy, 27

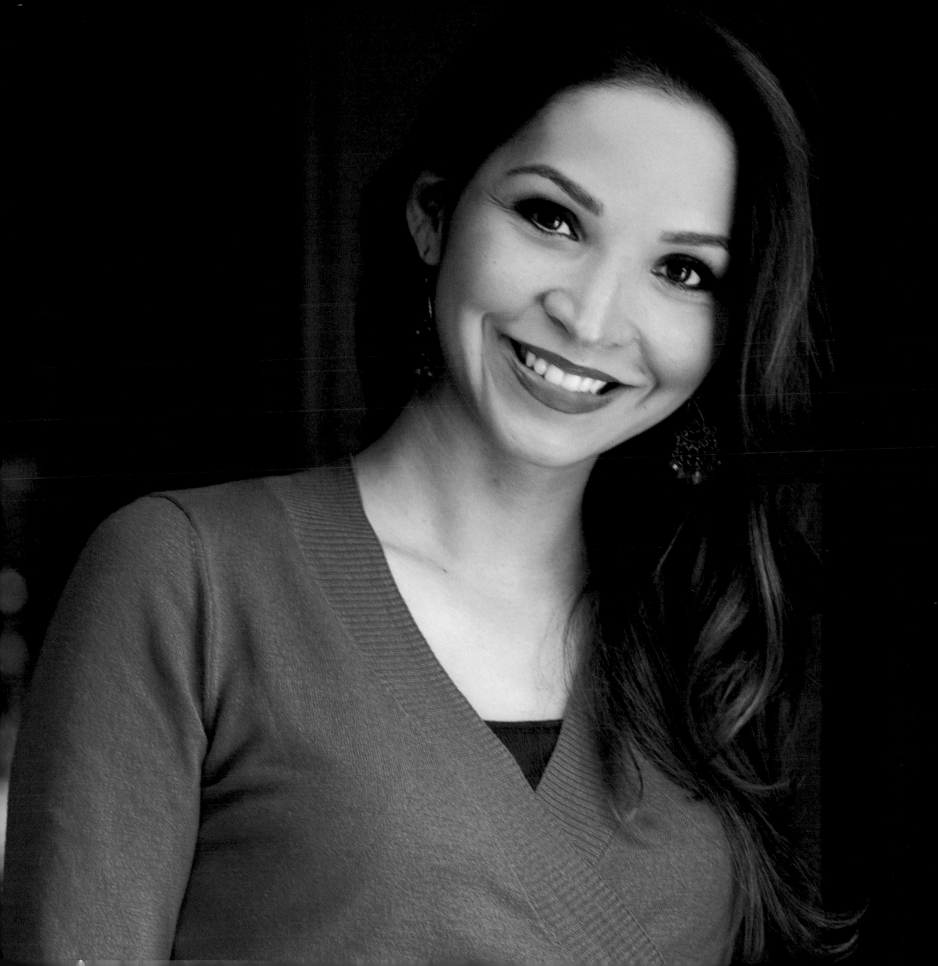

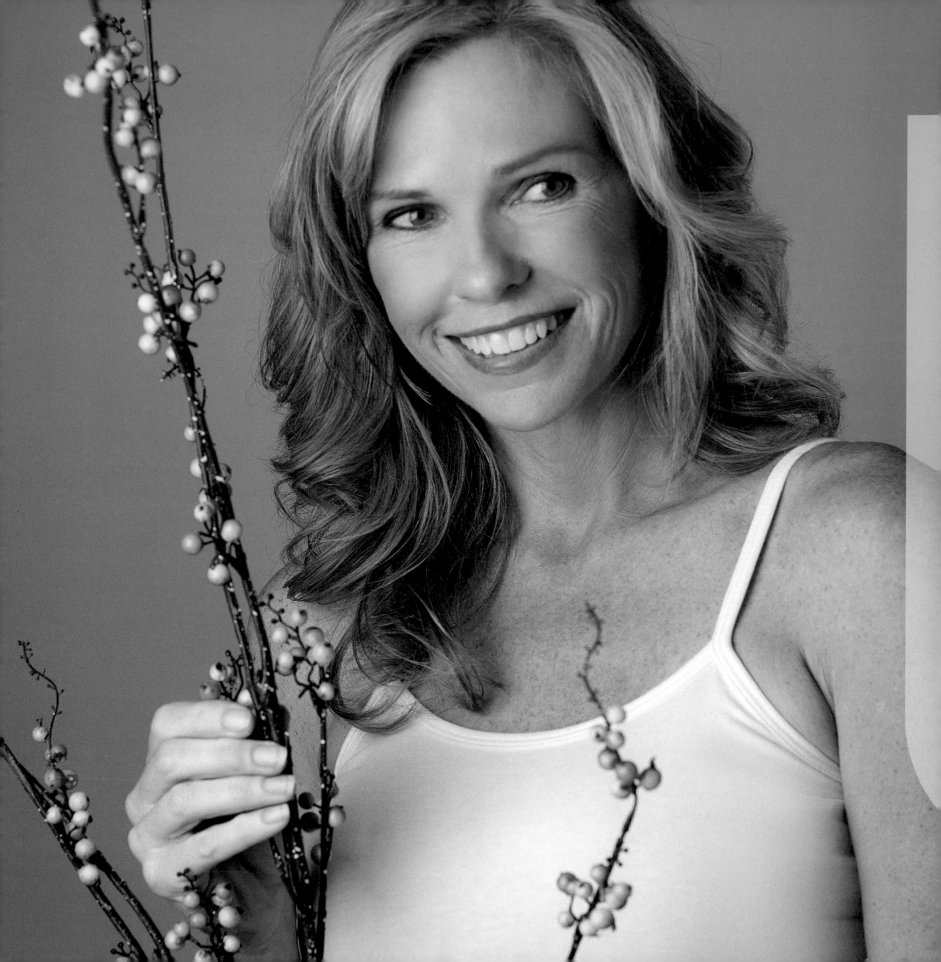

# CHAPTER 11

# PRODUCTS

> " Skin care has to be the number one priority to maintain A YOUTHFUL COMPLEXION."
>
> – Teri, 50

The marketing and sale of cleansers, moisturizers, cosmeceuticals, and cosmetics is a multi-billion-dollar industry. How do you navigate through the maze of products and promises? Which combination of potions and lotions is the real deal? In short, the answer depends on your age, skin type, pre-existing conditions, budget, and personal preference. This chapter will equip you with the tools needed to distinguish between proven products and hype.

# Why it is confusing

IT HELPS TO START BY FORMALLY DEFINING COSMETICS, DRUGS, AND COSMECEUTICALS SO WE CAN APPRECIATE THE DISTINCT NATURE OF EACH.

Cosmetics are products applied to the body to cleanse, beautify, promote attractiveness, or alter appearance. They do not require U.S. Food and Drug Administration (FDA) approval and can be purchased over-the-counter.

Drugs are products intended for treating or preventing disease and must undergo testing to get approval from the FDA. These include products such as tretinoin cream and tazarotene (Tazorac®) cream.

Cosmeceuticals are cosmetics that claim the action of a drug, such as restoring youthful appearance. Cosmeceuticals are not subject to FDA approval, and no testing is required. Technically they cannot claim drug-like action. Examples of cosmeceuticals are creams containing vitamins, lower-strength alpha hydroxy acids (AHA), and retinols. Cosmeceuticals may be sold over-the-counter or dispensed in a physician's office. Cosmetic dermatologists are familiar with the studies that have been performed and can help lead you toward products that will improve your skin.

## A conversation with the doctor

PATIENTS ALWAYS ASK WHICH PRODUCTS TO USE.

No one magic potion will stop aging and transform your appearance.

The products that will make a difference are not glamorous and include daily sunblock, a nightly topical retinoid, and a moisturizer. Whatever brand, consistency and smell you prefer, and will use every day, is the best choice for you. When choosing a product, look for ingredients proven to work and vehicles that are not irritating. If you are acne prone, make sure the product is labeled "non-comedogenic," which means it won't clog pores.

# Skin Deep

THERE ARE MULTIPLE LAYERS TO THE SKIN: THE EPIDERMIS, DERMIS AND FAT. Each layer plays a vital role in the appearance of healthy skin. The epidermis is the outermost layer. This is the area that is partially removed by exfoliation and microdermabrasion. Below the epidermis, the dermis contains collagen and elastic fibers. Over time sunlight, smoking, and pollution damage the collagen and elastic fibers, leading to wrinkles and sagging of the skin. The products mentioned in this chapter work by restoring the skin layers to their original thickness, organization, and content.

# What exactly should products do?

In general, cleansers degrease the skin and remove makeup. Some products also remove a few skin cells from the top layer of skin, which makes the surface smoother. Like the reflection off a granite countertop, light reflects off this smooth surface and the eye perceives an even, dewy, and healthy glow. However, too much glow is perceived as oiliness. Cleansers remove extra oil.

Moisturizers and anti-aging products try to restore the complex and perfectly balanced milieu of younger skin, hydrating the top layer of skin, and promoting new collagen growth below.

From a healthy skin perspective, makeup should not occlude hair follicles or irritate the skin. From a cosmetic standpoint, makeup colors and textures are chosen to enhance your individual features and mirror the colors seen in youthful faces.

# Product options and how they work

**CLEANSERS**: If you have sensitive skin or if you are less than 30 years old, your cleanser should simply remove makeup and excess grease.

Surfactants work by breaking up grease into smaller molecules so they can be washed away. This property makes your skin feel "clean," but you may perceive it as dry.

It's important to use a facial cleanser, not just your body bar soap. Facial cleansers are designed to be non-comedogenic, which means they do not clog pores. They usually contain moisturizers, so they do not dry delicate facial skin.

Avoid ingredients that cause stinging or irritation, like alcohol and menthol. Ingredients are listed on the bottle in order of greatest concentration to least. A product with alcohol listed last will be less irritating than one with alcohol listed first. Favorite gentle cleansers are Cetaphil®, CeraVe™, and Purpose®.

Additionally, if you are undergoing a laser treatment or chemical peel, you may want to consider cleansers designed for post-procedure skin. An example is SkinMedica®'s Sensitive Skin Cleanser.

If you have acne or oily skin and your skin is not sensitive, try a cleanser with salicylic acid or benzoyl peroxide like Neutrogena Oil-Free Acne Wash®, Clean & Clear Continuous Control Acne Wash®, or Proactiv® products. Your dermatologist can prescribe a cleanser with a higher percentage of these ingredients. Prescription formulas have better vehicles that may enable better delivery of the medication. Benzoyl peroxide bleaches towels and sheets, turning them white or pink. Use a white towel or place a towel over your pillow.

**TONERS**: Toners and astringents are optional. These products are alcohol-based. They have a drying effect to remove excess oil and tighten pores. Patients with rosacea, eczema, or dry skin should not use these products, as they will just further dry and irritate your skin. Patients with oily, acne-prone skin with large pores may like the feeling of a toner.

Constantly stripping oil from your skin may cause your skin to react by making more oil. Using a moisturizer regularly may actually make your skin less oily.

**MOISTURIZERS**: This is the MOST important part of any skin care regimen. Everyone, including teens and men, should use a facial moisturizer. Facial moisturizers are better than regular body lotions because they are formulated to be non-comedogenic. Some patients like thin moisturizers with a light feel, whereas others prefer thick creams that feel more occlusive. So pick your favorite, the one you will look forward to putting on twice a day. Lotions have more water than creams. Serums are somewhere in between. Unless your skin type is oily, opt for a serum or cream formulation.

▸ **Examples of thin moisturizers**: Cetaphil® lotion, Moisturel® lotion, CeraVe™ lotion, Clinique Dramatically Different Moisturizing Lotion®

▸ **Examples of thick moisturizers**: Cetaphil® cream, Olay Regenerist Daily Regenerating Serum®, Crème Ancienne™ by Fresh®

Adding sunscreen to moisturizer is a tricky science. Sunscreen makes some products more opaque, casting a whitish or bluish light on the skin. This happens more with physical sunscreens (zinc oxide, titanium dioxide, and iron oxide). If you are not allergic, try chemical sunscreens, which are less likely to change the consistency and color of the moisturizer. The American Academy of Dermatology recommends SPF 30 for daily use. Therefore, SPF 30 sunscreen should be applied under your makeup or moisturizer even if they contain a lower SPF, such as SPF 15.

▸ **Moisturizers with chemical sunscreens**: Neutrogena Healthy Skin® face lotion, Olay Total Effects 7X Visible Anti-Aging Vitamin Complex with UV Protection®, Clinique Super Defense Triple Action SPF 25®, Shiseido© Ultimate Sun Protection Cream, and CliniqueMedical®'s Daily SPF 38. Another potent UVA blocker is L'Oreal®'s line of products containing Mexoryl™ (Ecamsule), such as Revitalift® UV daily moisturizing cream with sunscreen.

▸ **Moisturizers with physical sunscreens**: Olay® (contains octinoxate, which is a chemical sunscreen with low allergy incidence), Blue Lizard Face® and Fallene Cotz® products. EltaMD Skincare™, sold in physicians' offices, has a combined physical/chemical sunscreen called UVFacial SPF 30+.

**PATIENT T!P**

Self-tanners are a safe and effective way to achieve a bronzed look. Remember that sunscreen should still be worn, as many self-tanning products do not contain SPF.

# Product options and how they work (continued)

**EXFOLIATING AGENTS**: Products like glycolic acid, salicylic acid, and physical exfoliators remove the topmost skin cells to reveal the newer skin cells below. These products are used in a variety of skin care lines to treat acne-prone skin. Examples include Glytone® and Neutrogena® Oil-Free Acne Wash. Glycolic acid and salicylic acid peels are also used by physicians to reduce the appearance of photoaging.

**ANTI-AGING PRODUCTS**: Who doesn't want a magic potion to turn back the clock? As a result, there is a growing multi-billion dollar industry that has developed products designed to fight the aging process.

The active ingredient in any anti-aging product has to be a retinoid. Retinoids, proven to soften fine lines, are vitamin A derivatives only available by prescription.

▸ **Retinoids and Retinol**: Retinoids come in creams, ointments, and gels. They are irritating at first, though most patients stop scaling after a month. Noticeable improvement will occur after three to six months of use. Some patients have little to no irritation with Renova®, a type of retinoid in a creamy soothing base. A popular retinoid, Tazorac® (tazarotene) is a potent formulation designed to improve acne lesions and scarring, as well as fine lines and wrinkles. Retinols are similar compounds available in over-the-counter products, yielding more modest effects. The Olay Professional ProX line of products is an over-the-counter anti-aging regimen containing antioxidants and retinol. They may take longer to reach a peak result. Avoid your eyes and eyelids.

**ANTIOXIDANTS**: Intuitively, one might expect that antioxidants slow the inflammatory reactions that break up collagen and age the skin. However, studies showing significant improvements are lacking, perhaps because it's difficult to get these ingredients to penetrate the skin. Still, antioxidants should help, and here's what we know so far.

▸ **Vitamin C (ascorbic acid)**: Sunlight creates inflammation mediated by free radicals, which can damage DNA and ultimately lead to collagen destruction and skin cancer. Vitamin C scavenges free radicals. It also plays an important role in collagen synthesis. It makes sense that topical vitamin C would combat skin aging, but vitamin C in cream formulation quickly breaks down and barely penetrates the skin surface. SkinCeuticals® has developed a serum vehicle for the preservation and delivery of vitamin C, called C E Ferulic®. They also make Phloretin CF™ which contains 10% L-ascorbic acid (vitamin C), 0.5% ferulic acid and 2% phloretin to inhibit UV-induced pigmentation and accelerate cell turnover.

# " Teri's story

I am a model and mother of six; three girls and three boys. I have been modeling since the age of 14, so taking care of my skin has always been very important to me. Skin care has to be your number one priority to maintain a youthful complexion. It doesn't matter what kind of great makeup you put on your face if you do not have good skin.

I learned good skin care at an early age, and I always find time to take care of my skin. I cleanse morning and evening, no matter how tired I am. After a moisturizing cleanser and alcohol-free toner, I apply a vitamin-enriched facial serum and moisturizer. In the morning, I add an additional sunblock of at least SPF 50. I do not drink alcohol, caffeine or smoke cigarettes. I get at least eight hours of sleep each night, run six miles every morning and eat healthy. By taking care of myself, I have always looked much younger than I am.

Because of my career, I have to be proactive in managing the effects of time and aging. My dermatologist recently prescribed a topical retinoid to use nightly to help maintain the benefits of my laser toning treatments. The first month I had blotchy red and dry areas, sometimes itching. But now, six months later, my skin has a radiant youthful glow and the fine lines have diminished. The pores seem a little smaller too. The results are wonderful."

AGE: 50
CONCERN: DULL SKIN
WITH FINE LINES
TREATMENT: TOPICAL RETINOID
DOWNTIME: NO DOWNTIME

BEFORE

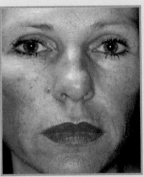

AFTER

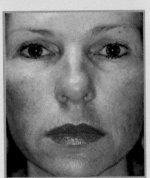

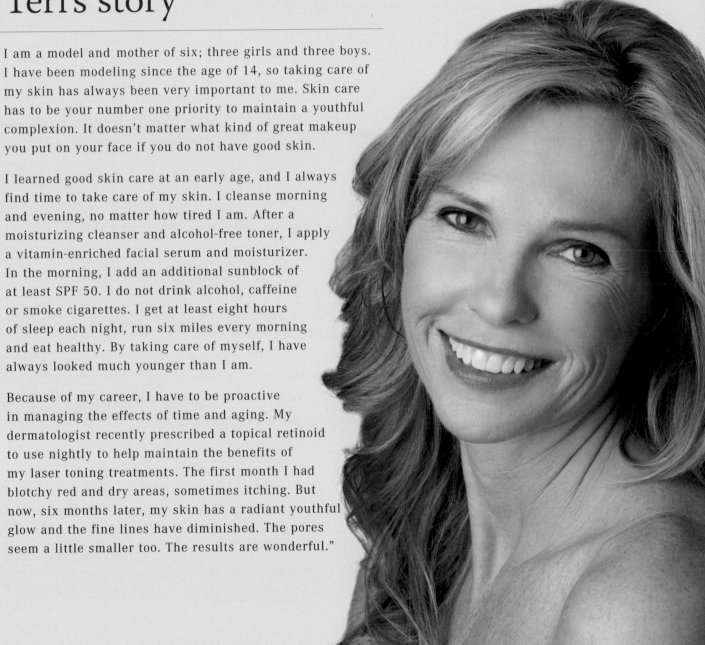

BEFORE

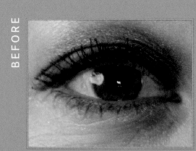

AFTER

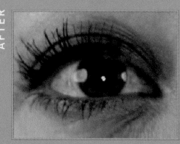

# Product options and
## how they work (continued)

**EYE MAKEUP AND BLUSH**: Here you are really choosing for color. Mix brands; try everything. From a dermatological standpoint, they're all the same—unless you're allergic. Itchy and dry eyelids are usually due to allergy. The most common eyelid allergens are nail polish and metals, like those in jewelry or eyeglass frames. There are hundreds of preservatives, vehicles, and fragrances in cosmetics that may also be the culprit.

If you are acne-prone, choose oil-free products labeled "non-comedogenic," which means it will not clog pores. If you are allergic, your dermatologist can do tests to identify the problem. If there is no allergy, have fun, and experiment.

**MAKEUP FOR CAMOUFLAGE**: To disguise imperfections, makeup such as Covermark® or Dermablend™ can be used to mask conditions such as vitiligo, birth-marks, burns, scarring, psoriasis, rosacea, eczema, and pigmentation.

**MICROSKIN™**: Microskin™ is a spray-on simulated skin which visually color-corrects to a patient's skin to cover various conditions, such as birthmarks or burns. Microskin™ can last up to several days on the skin and will gently wear off as the skin sheds. Microskin™ is new to the U.S. market and will be available at the Laser and Skin Surgery Center of New York. For more information, please go to www.microskin.com.au.

**EYELASHES**: There are several options available to promote darker, thicker, and longer eyelashes. Revitalash® is a product which is applied topically along the upper eyelid margin to promote longer lashes. Another similar topical treatment is Jan Marini's Marini Lash™. This eyelash conditioner contains peptides which promote eyelash and brow enhancement.

## " Kristel's story

As a dermatologist, I was excited to hear about Latisse® (bimatoprost ophthalmic 0.03% solution) when Allergan first launched this new topical medication to promote longer, thicker, and darker eyelashes. The clinical data show that after 16 weeks of nightly topical application with disposable applicators, lashes are 25 percent longer, 106 percent fuller, and 18 percent darker. Several of my colleagues were trying this medication, but I remained skeptical.

Being half Asian, I have always had sparse, straight eyelashes. I have tried numerous brands of mascara to lengthen the appearance of my eyelashes—from drugstore brands to department store products. If a topical product was marketed to improve eyelashes, I purchased it!

I had little luck with these products until recently, when I started Latisse®. After eight weeks of daily application, I noticed a difference in my eyelashes. I required less mascara, and it glided on smoothly. People stopped me at the grocery store or at work and asked what brand of mascara I used or if I was wearing false eyelashes. One patient told me that my eyelashes were the first thing she noticed about me! My eyelashes seem to brighten my eyes in photographs. I have had no adverse side effects with Latisse®. Some of the possible reported side effects include redness, itching of the eyes, or darkening of the iris, the colored portion of the eye.

Now that I've been on Latisse® for six months, I show my own before-and-after photos to my patients, who almost always ask for prescriptions immediately after I show them my results. I have written many prescriptions for Latisse®, and several patients have specifically asked for it. I feel confident recommending a product that works and will give patients their desired results."

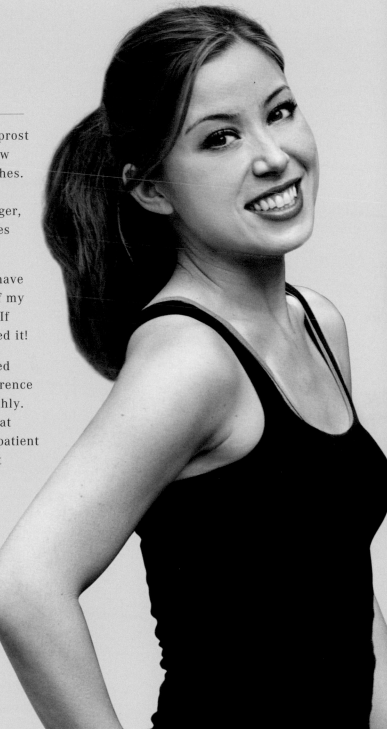

# Product options and
how they work (continued)

More recently, Latisse™ (bimatoprost ophthalmic solution 0.03%), marketed by Allergan®, was FDA approved for inadequate or sparse eyelashes. The medication is applied topically to the upper eyelid margin with a disposable applicator to make lashes darker, thicker, and longer. This product requires a prescription from your dermatologist or other healthcare provider.

**LIPS**: Think about your lower lip. It's always sticking out and exposed to sun. The central lower lip is a common place for skin cancers, and access to the many blood vessels in the lip makes them more likely to metastasize. Signs of too much sun exposure on the lip include brown spots and scaly, chapped areas, or blurring of the line between the lip and the skin. Choose a lipstick with SPF and reapply frequently. Clinique® makes a thick sunblock stick to stay put on lips.

Create the lip you want with makeup. Dot a lighter color, white, or shiny gloss on the center of your lower lip to create that full pout. Use a lip liner to feather a line at the edge of the lips, then blot your lips to avoid that harsh line. Remember the Cupid's bow is a cue for youth, so use liner to create definite angles at the center of your top lip (see right).

**CONCLUSION**: In summary, good skin requires maintenance. With the help of daily sunblock, a good moisturizer, and a topical retinoid, healthy skin has an even surface that glows. Cosmeceuticals and cosmetics can enhance the foundation achieved with a solid skin-care regimen and dermatologic procedures.

## Did you know?

THE CUPID'S BOW AND DEEP CREASE IN THE PHILTRUM ARE HALLMARKS OF A BABY. They are preserved throughout childhood and adolescence, fading with time. Use lip liner to recreate the definite edge between lip and skin, and the definite prominences that make up the Cupid's bow. If your lipstick gets stuck in the wrinkles, dermal fillers can be injected to fill out the lines and reclaim the prominent columns above the lip. Botox® removes the tiny lines around the mouth.

**Philtrum** is made of two vertical columns and a central depressed area.

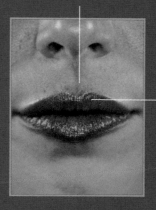

**Cupid's bow** is the upside-down W at the center of the top lip border. The angles of the W are sharp in youth.

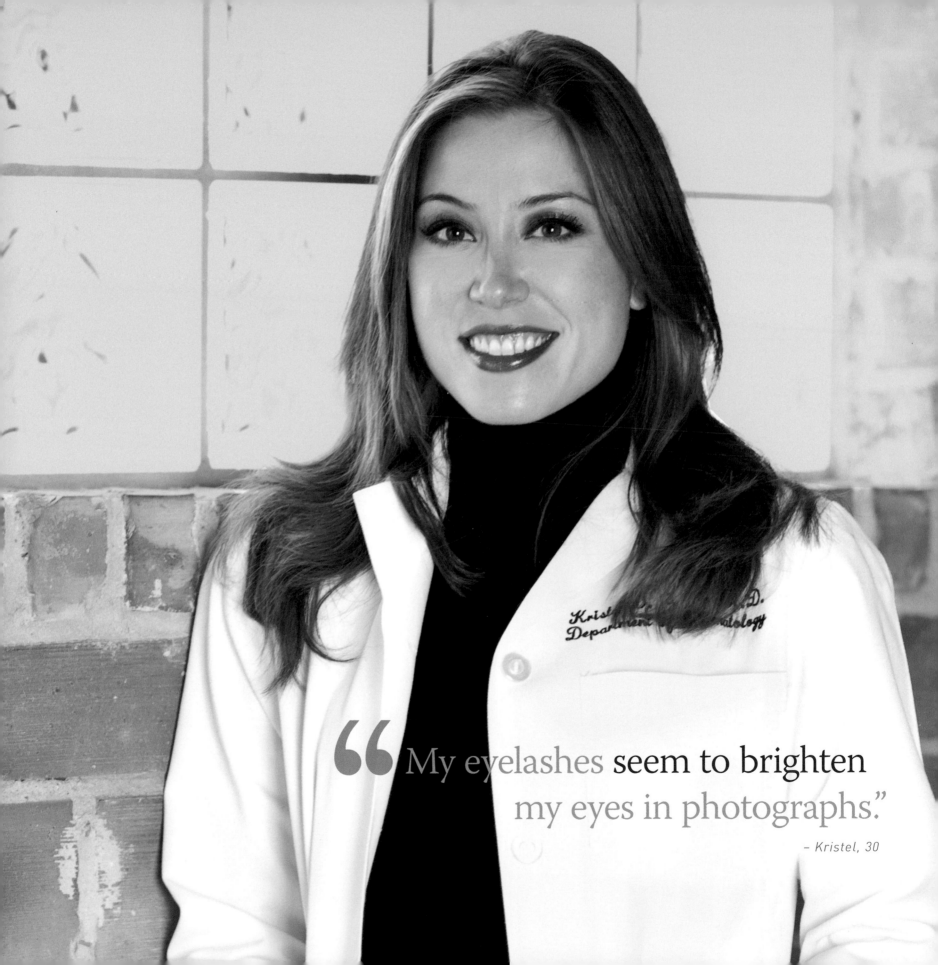

**"** My eyelashes **seem to brighten**
my eyes in photographs."

– Kristel, 30

> "By taking care of myself, I have always looked much younger than I am."
>
> – Teri, 50

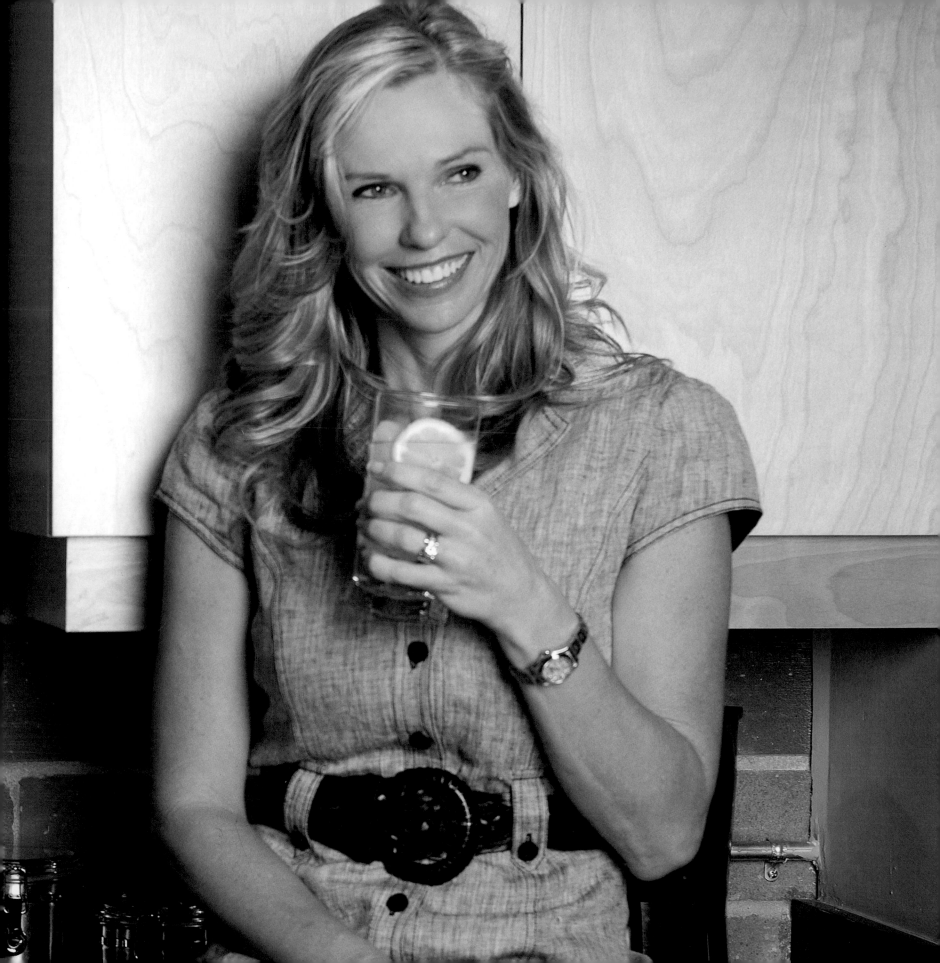

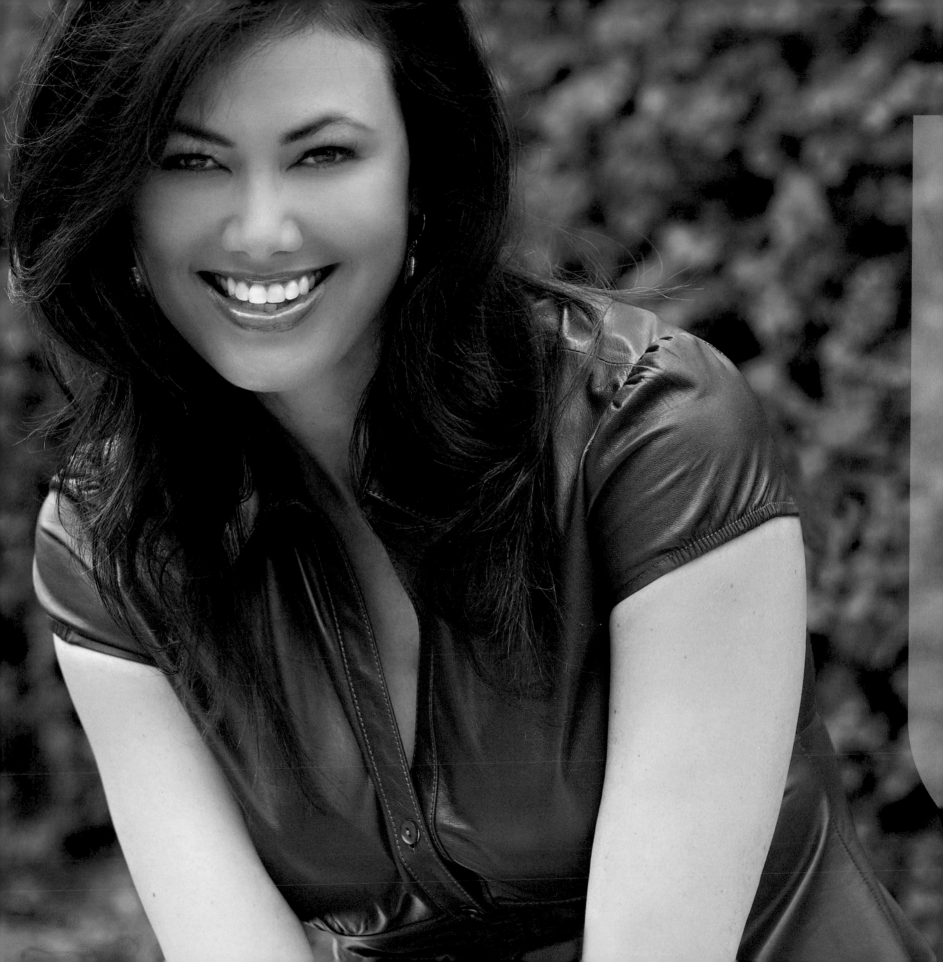

# CHAPTER 12

# CHOOSING A DOCTOR

" **Now I can laugh and joke** about the 'tiger stripes' that marked my face, BUT IT WASN'T FUNNY AT THE TIME."

– *Lucy*

Today's dermatologist has many options for improving skin complexion and skin conditions. In particular, cosmetic dermatologists have specialized training in skin aesthetic treatments.

A physician will be good at procedures he or she performs frequently. If you know exactly which procedure you want, seek a doctor with expertise in that particular area. If your doctor recommends a certain procedure, ask how many he or she has done.

“ It was a great feeling to have full confidence in how my wedding dress would look.”

*– Veronica, 29*

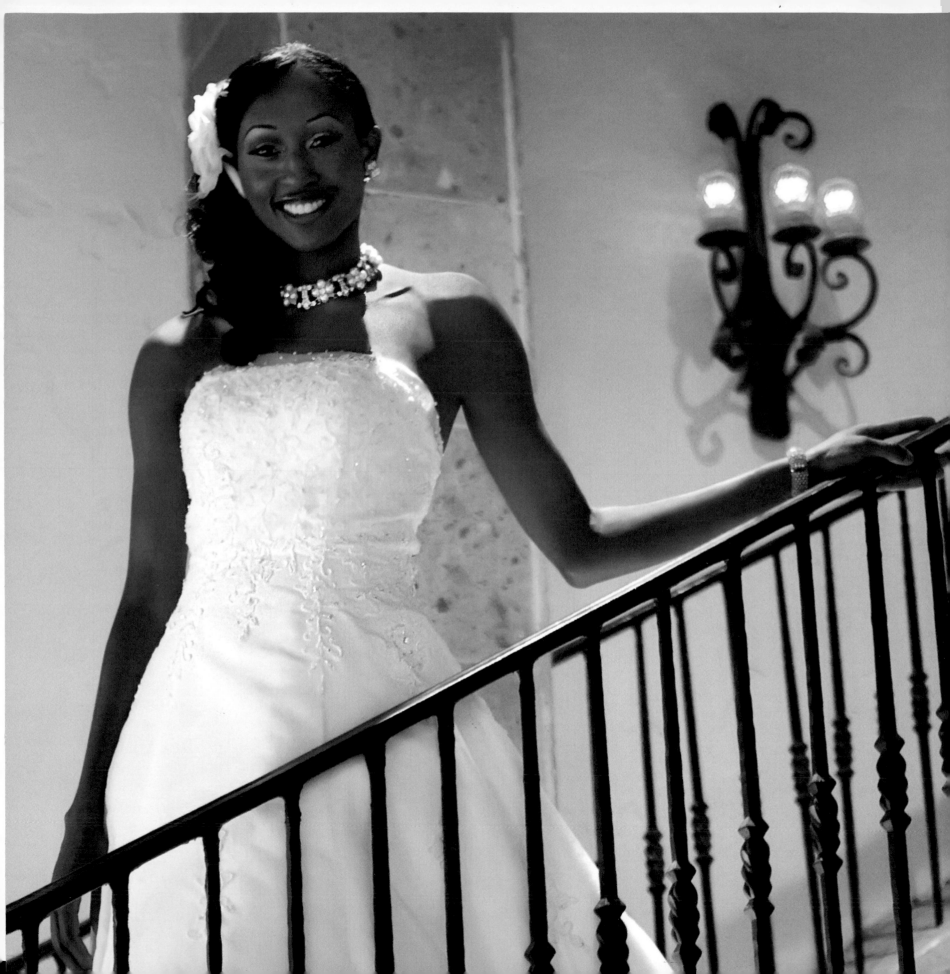